Dr Patrick Treacy was awarded 'Top Aesthetic Practitioner in the World' (2019) as well as 'Top Aesthetic Medical Aesthetic Practitioner UK & Ireland' (2019), earning himself a lifetime achievement place in the My Face My Body Aesthetic Medicine Hall of Fame. He was also given specialist research awards by both the British College of Aesthetic Medicine and the Irish Healthcare Awards, as well as a laureate from the Azerbaijani College of Aesthetic Medicine. He has been cited amongst the 'Ultimate 100 Global Aesthetic Leaders' for the past four years.

He is Chairman of the Ailesbury Humanitarian Foundation, previous Chairman of the Royal Society of Medicine Aesthetic Conference Committee (London) and serves on the editorial boards of six international aesthetic journals. Dr Treacy has written extensively about different cultures and their anthropology. He has worked with and written about the Kenyan Maasai, the Outback Australian Aboriginals and the Marsh Arabs in Iraq.

This book is dedicated to all the cherished souls we lost during the COVID-19 pandemic. To the friends, family members, colleagues, and acquaintances who succumbed to this relentless disease, you will forever hold a special place in our hearts.

Dr Patrick Treacy

PANDEMICS

And How They Change Society

AUSTIN MACAULEY PUBLISHERS™
LONDON * CAMBRIDGE * NEW YORK * SHARJAH

Copyright © Dr Patrick Treacy 2024

The right of Dr Patrick Treacy to be identified as the author of this work has been asserted by the author in accordance with sections 77 and 78 of the Copyright, Designs and Patents Act 1988.

All rights reserved. No part of this publication may be reproduced, stored in a retrieval system, or transmitted in any form or by any means, electronic, mechanical, photocopying, recording, or otherwise, without the prior permission of the publishers.

Any person who commits any unauthorised act in relation to this publication may be liable to criminal prosecution and civil claims for damages.

The medical information in this book is not advice and should not be treated as such. Do not substitute this information for the medical advice of physicians. The information is general and intended to better inform readers of their health care. Always consult your doctor for your individual needs.

A CIP catalogue record for this title is available from the British Library.

ISBN 9781398458185 (Paperback)
ISBN 9781398458192 (ePub e-book)

www.austinmacauley.co.uk

First Published 2024
Austin Macauley Publishers Ltd®
1 Canada Square
Canary Wharf
London
E14 5AA

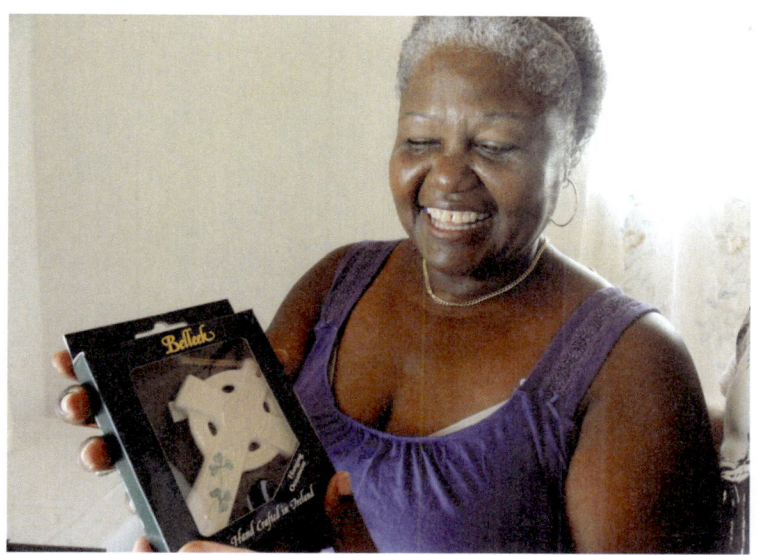

To those people like Brian Beardsley and Grace Dorcilien, whose laughter once filled the room, whose kindness knew no bounds, and whose presence brought joy to our lives, this book is a tribute to your memory. Your absence is deeply felt, but your spirit lives on in the memories we shared.

Table of Contents

Foreword   11

Viruses   19

    I Am the Poliomyelitis Virus and I Watched the Pharaohs Come and Go   27

    'The Russian Refugee Who Discovered the Polio Vaccine'   36

    I Am Flavivirus, Causer of Yellow Fever, and Who Held Up Construction of the Panama Canal.   39

    I Am the Variola Virus, Which Caused Smallpox, Once One of the Greatest Scourges of Mankind   48

    I Am the Ebolavirus, Which Caused Haemorrhagic Fever and Instilled Fear into the Heart of Africa   70

    I Am the Human Immunodeficiency Virus, Who Caused Worldwide Panic Before They Tamed Me   81

    I Am SARS-Cov-2, the Corona Virus, Who Caused the Worldwide Covid Pandemic   95

Bacteria   111

    I Am Bacillus Anthracis, 'Deliverer of the Jews to the Promised Land'   116

    I am *Yersinia Pestis*, Who Caused the Plague of Justinian and the Emergence of Christianity   133

    I Am *Yersinia Pestis*, Who Caused Typhus, the Emergence of Protestantism, and the Destruction of Napoleon's 'Grande Armee'   144

    I Am Mycobacterium Leprae, the Cause of Leprosy, and so Much Misery Worldwide   148

I Am *Mycobacterium tuberculosis*, and I Was with John Keats When He Died	156
I Am *Plasmodium Vivax*, Destroyer of the Roman Empire	169
I Am *Vibrio Cholerae*, and I Changed the World by Improving Sanitation	178
I Am *Treponema pallidum*, Who Sailed with The Slave Ships to America to Cause Syphilis	185
I Am *Cocoliztli,* and I Helped Wipe Out the Aztec Civilisation	194
References	**199**

Foreword

I am writing this foreword in isolation during lockdown in my Dublin home because of the SARS-CoV-2 pandemic now sweeping across the world. At the beginning of last year, we looked forward to the start of a new decade, and no one even knew that the corona virus or COVID-19 even existed. Now the virus has spread to almost every country, infecting over one hundred and thirty million people with nearly three million deaths. Infectious or transmissible diseases have existed since time immemorial, although the effect of pathogenic microbes in humans has become more problematic since man began farming and planted his food, most probably during the stone age. There is little doubt that the beginning of agriculture changed human history, but the epidemics that this domestication caused changed the social fabric of the society. History shows us that these pandemics often change the world for the better as they tend to shine a light on what is broken in our society and possibly also how to fix it.

The impact of pandemics on society can be both positive and negative, and it depends on various factors and contexts. Pandemics like COVID-19 have significant social, economic, and health consequences that can be challenging to manage. They can lead to a social and economic crisis, affecting societies and economies globally. The repercussions of a pandemic can be severe and far-reaching, impacting various aspects of life, such as employment, education, mental health, and social interactions. They cause great emotional distress as people witness illness and death among their community members. The fear and anxiety associated with the spread of a contagious disease can have a profound psychological impact on individuals and communities. The emotional distress caused by the COVID-19 pandemic in the UK has been significant. The pandemic has brought about various challenges, including health concerns, economic impact, social isolation, and disruption of daily life. Many individuals have experienced heightened anxiety, stress, and feelings of uncertainty due to the pandemic's widespread effects on society.

This was recently witnessed by the reaction of the British public to their previous Prime Minister, Boris Johnson. There have been reports and investigations suggesting that he misled Parliament on certain matters related to the COVID-19 pandemic. The UK Members of Parliament (MPs) recently voted to approve a report that recommended sanctioning Boris Johnson for lying to Parliament. The report highlighted instances where Johnson was accused of deliberately misleading Parliament regarding illegal COVID-19 lockdown parties that took place during his tenure as Prime Minister. We must also consider that pandemics can result in economic downturns, loss of income, and disruptions to industries and businesses.

Lockdowns, restrictions, and decreased consumer spending can lead to job losses, financial instability, and widening inequalities within societies. However, it's important to note that pandemics can also lead to positive outcomes, including strengthening public health systems: Pandemics often prompt a focus on improving public health systems, including disease surveillance, healthcare infrastructure, and research and development. These efforts can enhance preparedness for future health crises and lead to advancements in healthcare practices. They also accelerate scientific and technological advancements: The urgency to find solutions during a pandemic can drive scientific and technological innovations. This can include the development of vaccines, new treatment methods, and advancements in digital health technologies. They tend to increase social solidarity and resilience: Pandemics can foster a sense of solidarity and community resilience. People come together to support one another, show empathy, and implement collective measures to mitigate the spread of the disease. This can strengthen social bonds and build a sense of unity within society. Overall, while pandemics bring significant challenges and disruptions to societies, they also provide opportunities for growth, resilience, and progress in various aspects of public health, scientific research, and social cohesion Pandemics cause harm to societies, mainly because humans continually change their surrounding environment, as cities grow larger and take over territory previously inhabited by animals. Bacteria have been around for 3.5 billion years, viruses for 1.5 billion years and humans only for 130,000 years. Coronaviruses evolved about fifty million years or more, with the recent varieties estimated at about 8000 BCE, thereby implying quite a long period to coevolve with bat and avian species. Twentieth-century technology has led to improved travel, which means microbes can now travel around the world faster than ever.

Gone are the days when the voyage from England to India via the Cape of Good Hope with a regiment of soldiers took at least six months, and possibly another three or four months of traveling before they reached their final destination. Nowadays, a non-stop flight time from London to Mumbai takes about one seven hundredths of the time, around nine hours. Ever-expanding cities with larger populations mean respiratory viruses never have had it so good. The world was a vastly different place now than the first decades of the twentieth century. In this period, there were no public health systems and most doctors either worked for themselves or were funded by charities or religious institutions. It meant the people who spread diseases, either because of cramped living conditions or surviving on a poor diet were denied access to any health system at all. The privileged classes often looked down on the peasants and blamed their degeneracy on the cause of the illness, almost similar to the Church in the Middle Ages blaming the sick because God was punishing them as sinners. I witnessed this indifference by whites towards blacks with HIV in South Africa in the early nineties. In 2005, prevalence rates at antenatal clinics showed the disparity with only 0.6% of South African whites being HIV positive compared to 13.3% blacks. Many said, "it's a black person's disease," mainly because it quickly spread into the black communities by lorry drivers who used the services of prostitutes on the route from the copper mines in Zambia. 2005, prevalence rates at antenatal clinics.

There is evidence that whites totally disassociated themselves from black South Africans during the Spanish Flu in 1918, and this precipitated the first legislative steps towards apartheid. An estimated 500,000 people died in the 1918 flu pandemic in South Africa, the fifth hardest-hit country in the world. By the end of 1918, more than 127,000 Blacks and 11,000 Whites had succumbed to the epidemic. Hence, if we extrapolate these figures, probably 450,000 blacks had died before the pandemic ended. These people most probably became infected from ships bringing back members of the South African Native Labour Corps (SANLC) returning from France. Two ships, the *Jaroslav* and the *Veronej*, which arrived in Cape Town with members of the SANLC on board had docked at Sierra Leone, one of the places regarded as a central point of infection. Other historians say there were two waves, the first from the port of Durban, from where it spread to the rest of Natal and the Witwatersrand and the second spread from Cape Town harbour to the rest of the Cape, the Orange Free State, and the Western Transvaal. Not only did these people look down on the less fortunate as vectors of illness, but they also enacted health policies mainly geared to separating society into different e classes, without realising that this only helped to maintain and spread the illness back to them. Not only did they blame the people for their own illnesses, but as mentioned above, they were largely helped by a religious clergy who maintained it was due to the wrath of some God in the sky who was angry with their actions. This theory of disease asserts that pandemics and epidemics are really a punishment sent by an angry God for disobedience amongst his flock. The Church have used this superstitious nonsense to gain an upper hand during all of the previous pandemics (especially the Justinian plague!) and this was one of the reasons they encouraged the burning of libraries and did not want people to have a scientific education. Typhus and cholera ran rampant while priests sold indulgences to help get the dying into some supposed heaven in the sky.

The 'Spanish' flu claimed between 50 and 100 million lives, possibly five percent of the global population. Like the Justinian plague gave rise to Christianity, the bubonic plague brought an end to serfdom, the 'Spanish' flu in its wake, also brought massive social changes. The 1920s saw many governments embracing the concept of socialised medicine—it began with socialist Russia but quickly spread to France, New Zealand and eventually to Great Britain, although it took the hard-fought soldiers coming back from WW11 to force that politically. After the war, the growing influence of the United States and the fledgling World Health Organisation brought an end to the privileged classes and they set out ambitious fundamental rights of every human being without distinction to some level of proper health care. As we enter the final days of yet another global pandemic, nobody really knows what the future holds or whether the new vaccines will curtail the associated disease. The current COVID-19 pandemic will establish a major anchor point in the twenty-first century, curtailing our ability to travel to other nations. Since the initial HIV/AIDS pandemic started, I have visited most of the nations of central and eastern Africa in some humanitarian role and this is reflected in my previous books. However, it has given me the opportunity to write and contemplate on my life and travels to date, while also depriving me of previously arranged lecturing opportunities in Taipei, Monaco, and Toronto. These past years have been important for me, bringing me many accolades, and I was honoured to be voted Chairman of the Royal Society of Medicine Aesthetics Conference Committee (London). The MyFaceMyBody organisation gave me a specialist award for contributions to aesthetic medicine and I was given multiple awards for work related to my research into wound healing in many nations, including the United States, United Kingdom, Ireland, France, Mexico, Monaco, Azerbaijan, and Egypt.

People often ask, which was the worse period of all? American medieval historian Michael McCormick who chairs the Harvard University Initiative for the Science of the Human Past gives an interesting view. It wasn't 1349 when the Black Death wiped out half of Europe. Not even 1918, when the flu killed 50 million to 100 million people, mostly young adults. But rather 536AD. In that year, a mysterious fog encircled the earth, plunging Europe, the Middle East, and parts of Asia into darkness, day and night and it lasted for eighteen months. Summer temperatures in the summer of 536 AD fell 1.5°C to 2.5°C, starting the coldest decade on earth for over two thousand three hundred years. Without sunlight, crops failed and there was a famine in many European countries, including Ireland for the next three years. Snow fell during the summer months in China. The lack of sunlight caused vit D deficiencies and when the bubonic plague struck the Roman port of Pelusium, Egypt in 541AD, people had weakened immunity and what came to be called the Plague of Justinian spread rapidly, wiping out one-third to one-half of the population of the eastern Roman Empire and hastening its collapse. This also gave the Churches an opportunity to blame sinners as the cause, and a chance for them to create converts hoping that their intervention would somehow alleviate their symptoms. It is now thought that these 'Dark Ages' were actually due to a volcanic eruption in Iceland that spewed ash across the Northern Hemisphere early in 536. This was followed by two other eruptions in 540 and 547. The repeated volcanic eruptions followed by plague plunged Europe into an economic stagnation that lasted until 640. As mentioned, pandemics bring with them times of radical change in their wake. The necessity for remote consultations and healthcare delivery has accelerated the integration of technology into medical practice. Doctors are indicating that certain changes made during the pandemic are likely to be permanent. This includes an increased reliance on personal protective equipment (PPE), changes in patient flow and waiting room setups, and a continued emphasis on infection control measures. In the meantime, I will reflect on where I've been and am thankful to have experienced the imaginary world of my childhood. This book is dedicated to all the cherished souls we lost during the COVID-19 pandemic. To the friends, family members, colleagues, and acquaintances who succumbed to this relentless disease, you will forever hold a special place in our hearts. May this dedication serve as a reminder of the strength, resilience, and love that united us during these challenging times. Each page of this book is dedicated to the lives touched by the pandemic, an everlasting homage to your indomitable spirit and the profound impact you made. In honouring your memory, we strive to build a world that cherishes life, embraces compassion, and values the interconnectedness of our global community. May your legacy inspire us to be kinder, more empathetic, and united in our pursuit of a brighter future.

Though you are no longer physically with us, your presence endures in the stories, laughter, and love that will forever echo in our hearts. This book is dedicated to you, our beloved angels.

Prof, Dr Patrick Treacy
78 The Sweepstakes
Ballsbridge
Dublin D04XV66
June 2023

International Medical Awards 2019

- Winner – MyFaceMyBody 'Top Global Medical Practitioner' 2019 (Las Vegas) November 2019
- Winner – MyFaceMyBody 'Top UK & Ire Medical Practitioner' 2019 (Las Vegas) November 2019
- Winner – AMEC Anti-aging & Beauty Trophy 'Best Global Clinical Case' (Monaco), October 2019
- Winner – Irish Healthcare Award 'Best Medical Aesthetic Clinic' (Dublin), Sept 2019

International Medical Awards 2018

- Winner – MyFaceMyBody Specialist Award 'Scientific Contributions to the Aesthetic Industry' (London), March 2018

- Winner – Irish Healthcare Award 'Best Medical Research Award' (Dublin), March 2017
- Winner – MyFaceMyBody Award 'Ultimate 100 Global Aesthetic Leaders' (Los Angeles), August 2017
- Second – AMEC Anti-aging & Beauty Trophy 'Best Global Clinical Case in Laser Medicine' (Monaco), September 2017
- Second – AMEC Anti-aging & Beauty Trophy 'Best Global Clinical Case in Thread lifting' (Monaco), September 2017
- Winner – British College of Aesthetic Medicine 'Quality & Research Award'(London) September 2017
- Winner – AIDA Trophy 'Best Clinical Case in Aesthetic Medicine in Dermatology & Aesthetics' (Abu Dhabi) Oct 2017
- Winner – AAAMC Trophy 'Contribution to Development of Aesthetic Medicine' Azerbaijan Nat. Organizing Committee (Baku) Oct 2017
- Winner – John Bannon Award for the 'Best Clinic in Ireland' at the Aesthetic Awards (London), December 2017

International Medical Awards 2016-2017

- Winner – Irish Health & Beauty Award 'Best Cosmetic Surgery Clinic in Ireland 2016' (Dublin), June 2016
- Winner – 'Safety in Beauty Award Aesthetic Doctor of 2016' (Highly Commended) (London), June 2016
- Winner – AMEC Anti-aging & Beauty Trophy 'Best Clinical Research Case in Aesthetic Medicine' (Paris), September 2016
- Winner – CCME Mexican Congress Medal for 'Excellence in Medical Aesthetics' (Mexico), November 2016
- Winner – MyFaceMyBody Award 'Best medical research for wound healing' (London), November 2016

Viruses

What is a virus?

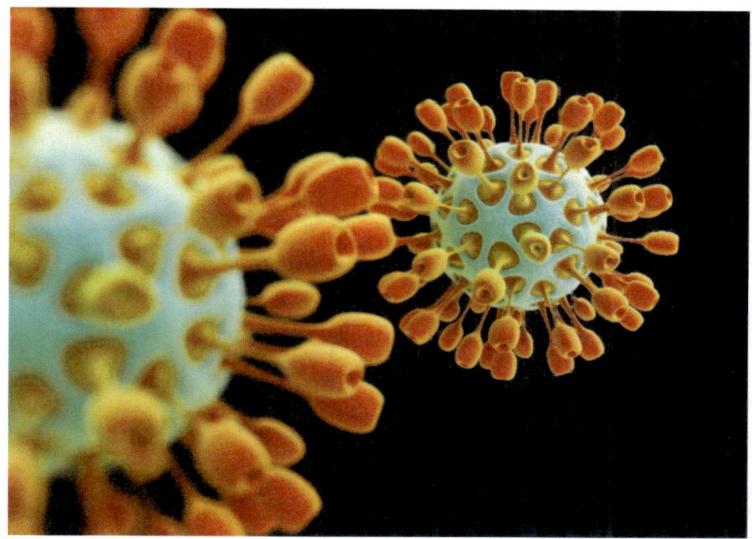

A virus is a fantastically small agent that can cause an infection and can only reproduce itself inside the living cells of another organism. They have the ability to grow in any ecosystem and infect not just humans but nearly everything on the planet with a reproductive ability from bacteria to animals. They are composed from short sequences of nucleic acid, which is a large molecule found in all living things and essential to store information of every living cell on Earth. They could be compared to a cassette tape, a CD or DVD that had the ability to make copies of itself. The two main classes of nucleic acids are deoxyribonucleic acid (DNA) and ribonucleic acid (RNA). The nucleic acid may be single – or double-stranded. Viruses are composed of short sequences of nucleic acid, either DNA or RNA wrapped in a protein shell. The protein shell is like the plastic cover on the outside of a DVD disc. Most music now is digitalised to prevent scratches or cracks, causing interference to the final copy. When this happens to viruses, we call it a mutation or variation. Viruses are spread in the human population by various means, including airborne particles, faecal-oral contact, clothing, insects, and contact with other animals (zoonosis). Small aerosol particles from a cough or sneeze can remain airborne for hours.

When were viruses discovered?

Because viruses are so small, we did not have the technology to see them until recently. Most virus species have virions too small to be seen with an optical microscope, as they are one-hundredth the size of most bacteria, and it required the invention of the electron microscope to see and study them. The shapes of these virus particles range from simple helical and icosahedral forms to more complex structures. The first viruses to be seen were the larger ones containing a head and a tail. The virus injected nucleic acid into the other living cells through the tail. These larger ones infect bacteria and were called bacteriophages. Consequently, some countries, especially the Soviet Union.

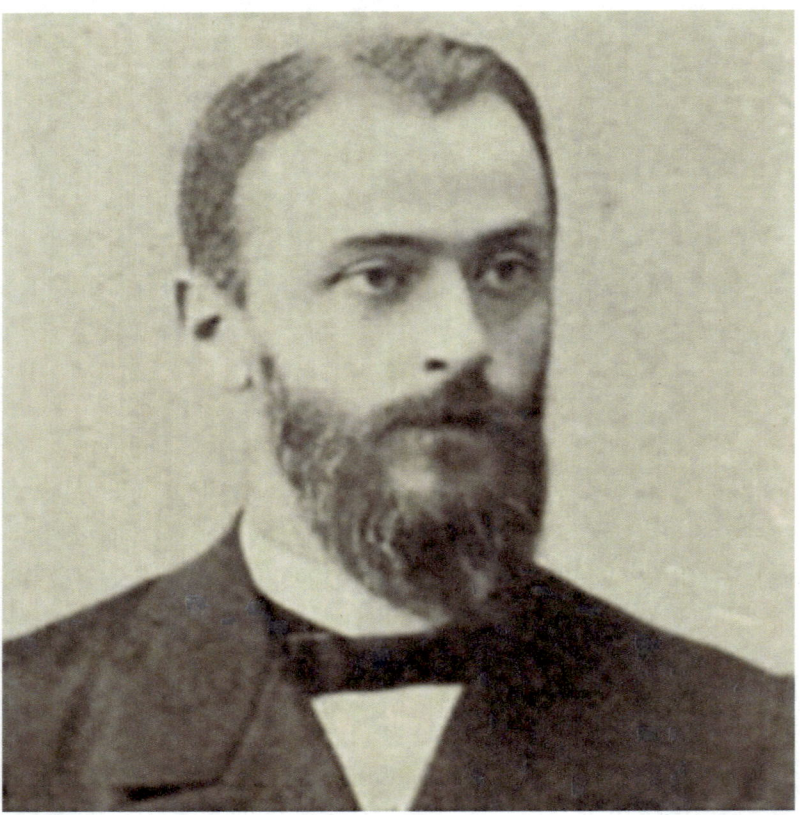

Dmitri Ivanovsky helped discover viruses and France deployed them to kill bacteria instead of using antibiotics. The viruses that infect humans or animal are a different shape, usually spherical or even rod-shaped to allow a key on their outside to attach to a lock on the cell that they want to invade. When infected, a host cell is forced to rapidly produce thousands of identical copies of the original virus.

In 1892, Dmitri Ivanovsky, a Russian microbiologist, conducted experiments on tobacco plants infected with tobacco mosaic disease. He filtered the sap from the diseased plants to remove bacteria, expecting that this would eliminate the infectious agent. However, he found that even after filtration, the filtered sap retained its ability to infect healthy tobacco plants. This observation led Ivanovsky to conclude that there must be an unknown, filterable pathogen causing the disease. This experiment played a crucial role in the discovery of the first virus, the tobacco mosaic virus.

In 1898, a Dutch microbiologist, Martinus Beijerinck called the filtered, infectious substance a 'virus' and this discovery is the beginning of virology. Beijerinck said the infectious material had to be smaller than a bacterium and called it a virus. He was the first to recognize that viruses are reproducing entities that are different from other organisms. He also discovered new types of bacteria from soil but did not communicate properly with other scientists of the day, particularly Robert Koch, turning down an invitation to visit his laboratory. Since Ivanovsky's article describing a non-bacterial pathogen infecting tobacco plants more than 6,000 virus species have been described in detail of the millions of types of viruses in the environment. Beijerinck was born on March 16, 1851, in Amsterdam, Netherlands, and passed away on January 1, 1931, in Gorssel. He is recognized as one of the pioneers in the field of virology and is considered a founder of the field of general microbiology. Beijerinck made significant contributions to the understanding of viruses, specifically through his work on tobacco mosaic disease. In 1898, he formulated the concept of a virus as an infectious agent that could only replicate within a living host cell. His experiments and observations laid the foundation for the field of virology and provided crucial insights into the nature of viral infections. Throughout his career, Beijerinck conducted extensive research on various topics, including microbiology, botany, chemistry, and genetics, authoring over 140 scientific papers. His contributions and discoveries significantly advanced our understanding of microorganisms and their role in the natural world.

What are viruses made from?

Viruses are effectively a collection of four molecules, proteins, nucleic acids, lipids, and carbohydrates, but on their own they can do nothing until they enter a living cell. Without cells, viruses would not be able to multiply. Therefore, viruses are not living things as only in their host's nucleus can they find the machines, proteins, and building blocks with which they can copy their genetic material before infecting other cells. The simplest viruses contain only enough RNA or DNA to encode four proteins. These proteins interact to cause viruses to self-assemble as a result of interactions to form a viral capsid, which interacts with the nucleic acid to form new viruses to lyse the host cell and spread to neighbouring cells to continue the cycle. Studies of viral replication indicate that most viruses are made of either two or three parts. All include genes. These genes contain the encoded biological information of the virus and are built from either DNA or RNA. All viruses are also covered with a protein coat to protect the genes. When not inside an infected cell or in the process of infecting a cell, viruses exist in the form of independent particles, or virions. The entire infectious virus particle, called a virion, consists of the nucleic acid and an outer shell of protein. A virion has an outer protein case (capsid) and an inner core of nucleic acid (either ribonucleic or deoxyribonucleic acid—RNA or DNA). One could say that the inner core gives the virus its infectivity, and the outer capsid provides us with details of its type (specificity). Claverie suggested that the viral factory corresponds to the organism, whereas the virion is used to spread from cell to cell.

Are viruses alive?

The question of whether viruses are alive is a topic of debate among scientists. Viruses are unique entities that exhibit some characteristics of life but lack others. They are considered to be on the boundary between living and non-living entities. Some biologists consider viruses to be a life form because they carry genetic material, reproduce, and evolve through natural selection but most say viruses are not alive as they do not carry out respiration, they are not made out of cells, they do not require nutrient to grow, they cannot synthesise proteins and they cannot make their own energy. Viruses are acellular, meaning they do not have cells. They consist of genetic material, either DNA or RNA, encased in a protein coat called a capsid. Some viruses also have an outer envelope. Viruses cannot carry out essential life processes such as metabolism and reproduction on their own. They require a host cell to replicate and produce new viral particles. Viruses appear to have functions, different in nature but comparable in complexity to bacteria. As they do not grow or increase in biomass in the normal way, they tend to remain the same size and simply replicate by hijacking all the machinery within another cell. While viruses can undergo evolution and adapt to their environments, they lack the ability to reproduce independently. They rely on host cells to provide the necessary machinery for replication. Additionally, viruses do not display characteristics commonly associated with living organisms, such as cellular structure, growth, and response to stimuli. They cannot carry out their life-sustaining functions or reproduce without a host cell. Technically they lack ribosomes, minute particles consisting of RNA and associated proteins that function to synthesise proteins. They must use the ribosomes of their host cells to translate viral messenger RNA into viral proteins, which are needed for many cellular functions. Even though they definitely replicate and adapt to their environment, viruses are more like androids than real living organisms. At a basic level, viruses are proteins and genetic material that survive and replicate within their environment, inside another life form. In the absence of their host, viruses are unable to replicate, and many are unable to survive for long in the extracellular environment. In conclusion, viruses are considered to be non-living entities because they lack the ability to carry out essential life processes on their own. However, they possess some characteristics of life and have a significant impact on living organisms as agents of infection and disease.

How do viruses spread?

Viruses can spread through various mechanisms. The most common methods of virus transmission include:

- Droplet transmission: This occurs when an infected person coughs, sneezes, talks, or breathes, releasing respiratory droplets containing the virus into the air. These droplets can then be inhaled by nearby individuals, leading to infection. This is a common route of transmission for respiratory viruses like influenza and COVID-19.
- Direct contact: Viruses can spread through direct physical contact with an infected person. This can happen through activities such as shaking hands, hugging, or touching surfaces contaminated with the virus and then touching the face, mouth, or eyes.

- Indirect contact: Indirect contact occurs when a person touches a surface or object contaminated with the virus and then touches their face, mouth, or eyes, allowing the virus to enter their body.
- Airborne transmission: Some viruses can remain suspended in the air for extended periods and be inhaled by individuals in the vicinity. This mode of transmission is more relevant to certain respiratory viruses like measles and tuberculosis.
- Vector-borne transmission: Certain viruses are transmitted by vectors such as mosquitoes, ticks, or other insects. These vectors act as carriers, transmitting the virus from one host to another through bites.

It's important to note that the specific mode of virus transmission can vary depending on the virus in question. Public health measures, such as vaccination, hand hygiene, wearing masks, and practicing respiratory etiquette, can help reduce the spread of viruses.

An air purifier with a HEPA may trap any airborne viruses, including the COVID-19 coronavirus, that happen to pass through it. Researchers have developed CRISPR-Cas13 enzyme-based technology that can be programmed to both detect and destroy RNA-based viruses in human cells. Researchers have turned a CRISPR RNA-cutting enzyme into an antiviral that can be programmed to detect and destroy RNA-based viruses in human cells.

I Am the Poliomyelitis Virus and I Watched the Pharaohs Come and Go

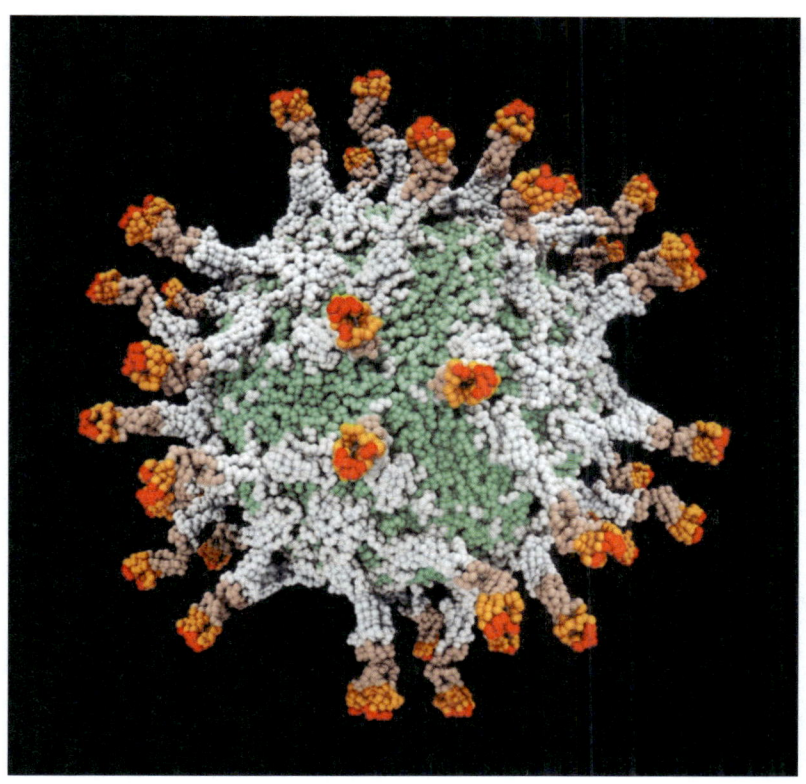

Poliomyelitis virus

Poliomyelitis is a highly infectious disease caused by a virus belonging to the Picornaviridae family. It is a viral infection that primarily affects the nervous system and is transmitted from person to person, mainly through the faecal-oral route. This means the virus enters the body through the mouth and spreads through contact with contaminated faeces, food, or water.

The clinical features are varied ranging from mild cases of respiratory illness, gastroenteritis, and malaise to severe forms of paralysis. Most people infected with the poliovirus do not experience any symptoms. The infection can occur without symptoms, mild illness (abortive poliomyelitis), aseptic meningitis (nonparalytic poliomyelitis). However, in some cases, the virus can invade the nervous system and cause paralysis, particularly in the muscles of the limbs. This condition is known as paralytic polio. The symptoms of paralytic polio can include fever, fatigue, headache, muscle pain, stiffness, and weakness. In severe cases, it can lead to permanent disability or even death if the muscles involved in breathing are affected. Polio primarily affects children under the age of 5. However, it can affect individuals of any age. Before the development of polio vaccines, polio was a widespread and highly feared disease, causing significant outbreaks and epidemics.

Scientists in the 1900s, established the genomic structure of the virus and doctors like Salk and Sabin discovered the oral polio vaccine (OPV) and the inactivated polio vaccine. Vaccination has played a crucial role in controlling and reducing the incidence of polio worldwide. The oral polio vaccine (OPV) and the inactivated polio vaccine (IPV) are the two types of vaccines used to prevent polio. Thanks to extensive vaccination efforts, the global incidence of polio has significantly decreased. In fact, polio cases have been reduced by over 99% since the launch of the Global Polio Eradication Initiative in 1988. However, the disease is still present in a few countries, and ongoing vaccination campaigns are necessary to achieve complete eradication.

Here is the story of the polio pandemic told from the virus's point of view

I am the Poliomyelitis virus, and I have inhabited this planet for many years than I care to remember, being transmitted by faecal-oral contamination, when someone eats contaminated food and water or touches objects where I have been. I can also spread from person to person through the mucous when somebody coughs or sneeze. I was there with the ancient Egyptians long before Menes united the two kingdoms of Lower and Upper Egypt in 3100BC. In fact, the finding of misshapen bones of some mummies show I was already celebrating my sixth hundredth birthday before his unification party. Usually, I multiply in the tissues of the throat or sometimes the mucosa of the lower gastrointestinal tract and stay there from one to three weeks. However, I tend to release my young a few days before symptoms start and continue an additional one week. In most cases, I cause no problems, maybe a flu-like illness, but in a small percentage, paralysis of their limbs can occur.

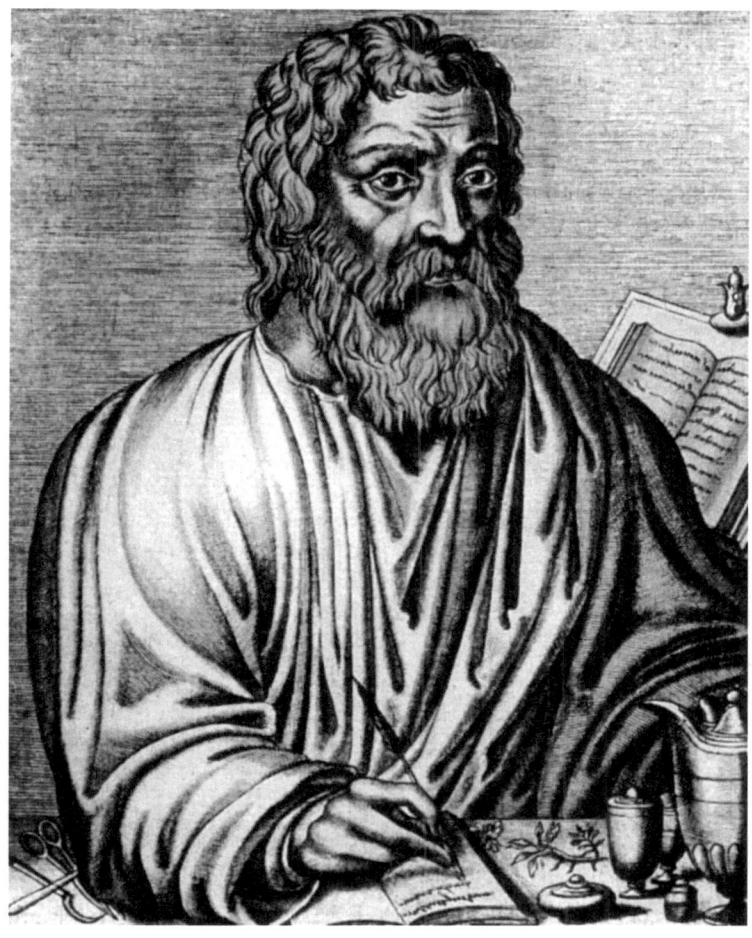

HIPPOCRATES – Greek physician c 460–377 B

But enough of that, suffice to say I must have liked the sunsets over the Nile because I was still there if you look at the stone reliefs of 1500 BC, those poor priests with their atrophied short legs, their muscle wasting, their crippled bone growth. Just look a little closer at the artefacts on show the next time you are down near that old sandy museum in Maydan El Tahrir, Cairo and you will probably see my calling cards. Anyway, having enough of the Akhenatens and the Amarnas, I decided I needed a Greek holiday and arrived on the island of Kos. It was just about the beginning of the fourth century, the time Ictinus was designing the Parthenon and Pericles was being proclaimed by Thucydides, as 'the first citizen of Athens'.

Well, who did I run into but the great Hippocrates himself and he even mentioned me under the title of 'infant paralysis' in his latest book 'The Hippocratic Corpus' OK! It wasn't exactly a bestseller, but with Plato, Philolaus and that newcomer Lysis of Epaminondas all trying to make the Christmas list, well he had some stiff opposition, you know. By the way, my name is Greek, pilios (gray), myel (marrow) and itis (inflammation).

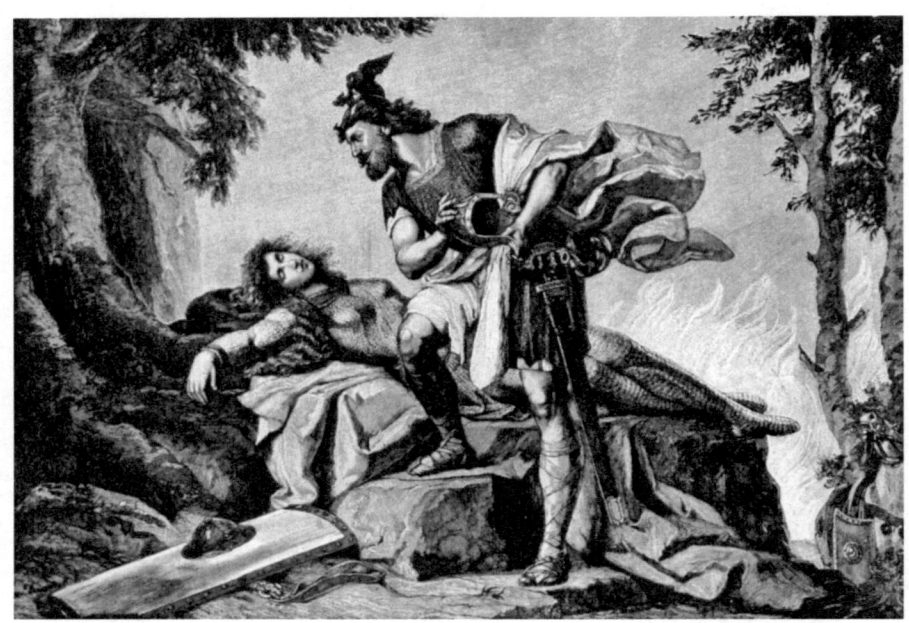

Siegfried awakens Brunhild, a scene from Wagner's Ring

And as the Roman Empire fell, and unwashed barbarians descended upon their cities, looting artefacts, and burning books, I went with the Irish who took up the great labour of copying all of Western literature and the Celtic physicians called me 'the pestilence that is called lameness'. For centuries, I remained a mild disease often ignored by physicians until some bright spark abandoned the chamber pot for the modern flush toilet and unwittingly transformed me into a paralysing agent of epidemic proportions. The improvements in the waste disposal and the widespread use of indoor plumbing during the late nineteenth century meant that babies were no longer exposed to me at a young age and acquired no natural immunity. So, many years later, when I visited the Scottish poet, Sir Walter Scott, still at the tender age of eighteen months, his doctors thought he had 'teething fever'. His medical grandfather, a gentleman called Dr Rutherford even suggested that they should take the boy out into the country where the clean air would be good for his lame leg.

I visited Stuttgart in 1840 and even got mentioned in a book by the renowned physician of the day, Dr Jacob von Heine. They later even called me the Brunhild virus meaning of course 'fighter in armour' but really being named after an Icelandic queen from the epic Nibelungenlied.

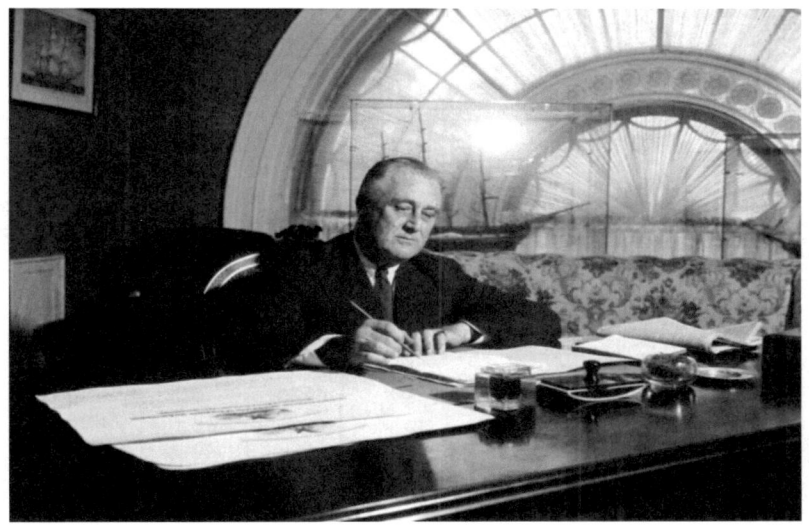

President Franklin Roosevelt signs bills in the East Hall of the White House on June 8, 1936.

Before global health initiatives, I left about 1 in 200 with permanent paralysis. I had a few brothers and one of them is rather wild, but they were all eradicated in 2015. I have been responsible for the majority of the world's paralytic polio cases before these vaccines became widespread. There were 350,000 cases of endemic poliomyelitis spread across 125 countries in 1988. Anyway, back to my tale. In 1916, I crossed the Atlantic and while poor Dubliner, Padraig Pearse was busy battling it out in the General Post Office as part of the Easter Rising, I checked out the new flushing toilets in New York. That summer I befriended thousands of young children in the city and panic erupted as thousands of families fled from Manhattan. Talk about bioterrorism at its best, the Department of Health quarantined the city and hundreds of families were turned back on Brooklyn Bridge. By the end of the summer, two thousand Manhattan children were dead and I had paralysed nine thousand others. By the time of the Great Depression, I was the most feared disease known on the planet and everywhere there was sanitation there were people hobbling around on crutches, rolling about in wheelchairs, lying immobile in giant iron lungs, the legions of sufferers, none knowing what was causing their affliction. Things got so bad that President Franklin Roosevelt actually declared a war on me and put the tremendous resources of post-war America in trying to develop a vaccine against me.

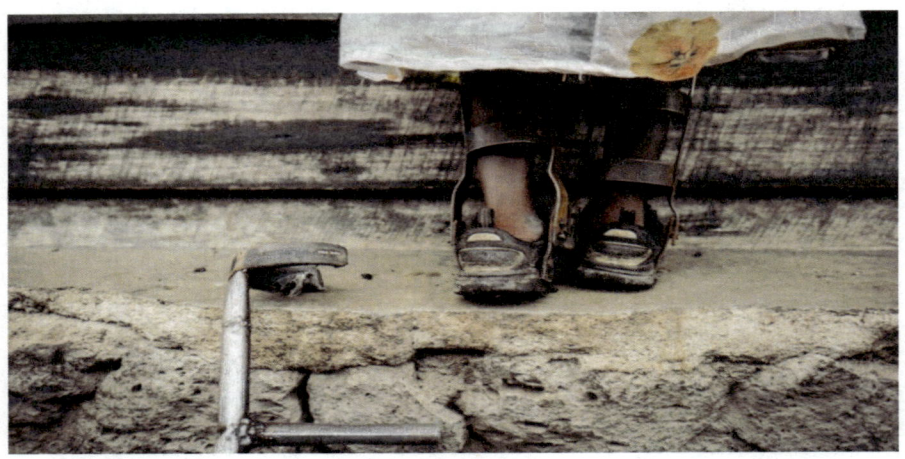

An 8-year-old girl fitted with callipers by an NGO in Goma, DRC

However, the 1930s, were years of great poverty and medical advances were often rushed in an effort to stop my advances. In 1935, field trials for a new vaccine were tried by Maurice Brodie and John Kollmer. Brodie concocted his vaccine from an emulsion of the ground-up spinal cords of infected monkeys. He even attempted to deactivate me by exposing me to formalin and then he tried the concoction on twenty monkeys and 3000 children. The less said about this the better as in the words of a historian of the period, "Something went terribly wrong, and his concoction was never used again."

Kollmer then tried mixing me with various chemicals and putting me in a fridge for two weeks. The new 'attenuated' virus, he called me. Well, he tried out this veritable 'witches brew' on a few monkeys, himself, his children, and twenty-two others. He even started to distribute it to hundreds of physicians across the country but after he was blamed for causing many cases of polio, some even fatal, he gave up the quest. Kolmer addressed a meeting of the Southern Branch of the American Public Health Association in 1935, with the words "Gentlemen, this is one time I wish the floor would open up and swallow me." To be fair, he did manage to pick up the pieces and go on to a successful, if not distinguished, research career. But poor old Brodie, he died shortly afterwards but not before accepting a minor research position in Michigan. It is rumoured in many circles that he took his own life, but either way he was not around to see Jonas Salk having a little more success with the problem. True, he also dipped me in formaldehyde, but he also heated me up in an effort to find my weak spot. You would have thought that after all those summers in Egypt and Greece, I would have been a bit more used to the heat, but as an American bomber with a Taliban in his sights, he knew that he had me on my back. In 1952, he inoculated his wife, and their three sons with his mixture and they all began producing antibodies to the disease, yet no one became ill.

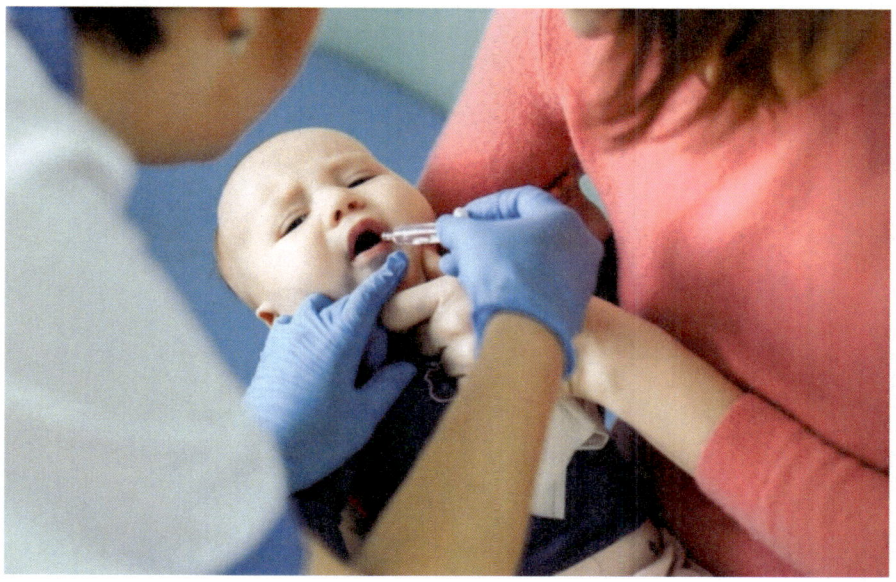

Sabin's vaccine on sugar

The following year he published the results in the Journal of the American Medical Association, and nationwide testing was carried out. By 1952, I had befriended over 57,628 cases, making it the worst year yet. His former mentor Thomas Francis Jr., who had helped him develop the influenza vaccine during the Second World War decided that America should start a mass vaccination of their schoolchildren. In the early 1960s, I was on the run and when Albert Sabin started to produce different oral versions of me, I decided to go into hiding. By 1964, approximately 100 million Americans had taken Sabin's vaccine on sugar cubes or sweetened syrup. The fact it could be taken orally and kept in the refrigerator until administration time meant it was easy to administer in third-world countries such as Africa. After taking the vaccine, you could even excrete live poliovirus from your faeces and immunise all your neighbours secondhandedly. What chance did I have! God bless the Jews for their ingenuity!

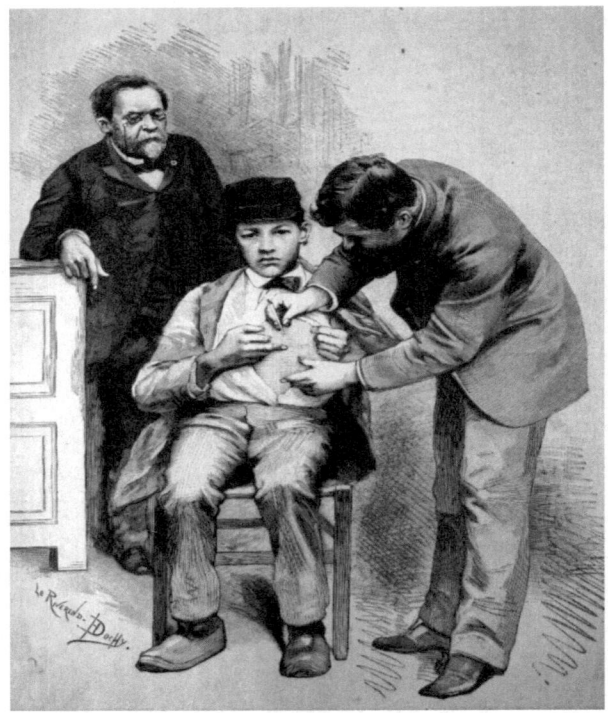

Injecting a boy at Pasteur's Laboratory

On July 6, 1886, nine-year-old Joseph Meister and his mother appeared at Pasteur's laboratory. Two days earlier, the young boy had been bitten repeatedly by a rabid dog. He was so badly mauled that he could hardly walk. His mother appealed to Pasteur to treat her son. Pasteur, after much trepidation, decided to treat the youth. Meister made a perfect recovery and remained in fine health for the remainder of his life. Pasteur became a hero and a legend. Rabies was the last major research of the great scientist. His health was failing and a paralysis of his left side from a serious stroke; he suffered in his 46th year made his working in the laboratory increasingly difficult. Pasteur died in 1895 after suffering additional strokes. Few people have contributed so much to medical knowledge as this great scientist.

****

In a tragic footnote to history, Joseph Meister, the first person publicly to receive the rabies vaccine, returned to the Pasteur Institute as an employee where he served for many years as gatekeeper. In 1940, forty-five years after his treatment for rabies that made medical history, he was ordered by the German occupiers of Paris to open Pasteur's crypt. Rather than comply, Joseph Meister committed suicide.

Soon I was only a memory in most of the industrialised world and the economic and social impact was incalculable, except for the makers of crutches, wheelchairs, and iron lungs who quickly went out of business or started work on drones that could be later used in Afghanistan. More recently the World Health Organisation took umbrage against me and said they would smoke me out and run me off the planet by 2005. In 1999, there were 7141 cases worldwide and this had dropped to 3500 in 2000, a 99% decrease from the 350 000 annual cases estimated in 1988. Last year 550 million children under five years were immunised and this included India, where 152 million children were vaccinated in three days. Following the widespread use of the poliovirus vaccine in the mid-1950s, new cases of poliomyelitis declined dramatically in many industrialized countries. A global effort to eradicate polio began in 1988, by the World Health Organization, and UNICEF. These efforts have reduced the number of cases diagnosed each year from 350,000 cases in 1988 to a low of 483 cases in 2001 (99.9 percent). In April 2012, the World Health Assembly declared that the failure to completely eradicate polio 'must not happen'. In 2015, polio was believed to remain naturally spreading in only two countries: Pakistan, and Afghanistan.

'The Russian Refugee Who Discovered the Polio Vaccine'

Albert Bruce Sabin was born in Bialystok Russia, (now a part of Poland) in 1906, the same year that one thousand people were killed in the San Francisco earthquake. His family were poor Jews and were persecuted by the horrific pogroms of the period.

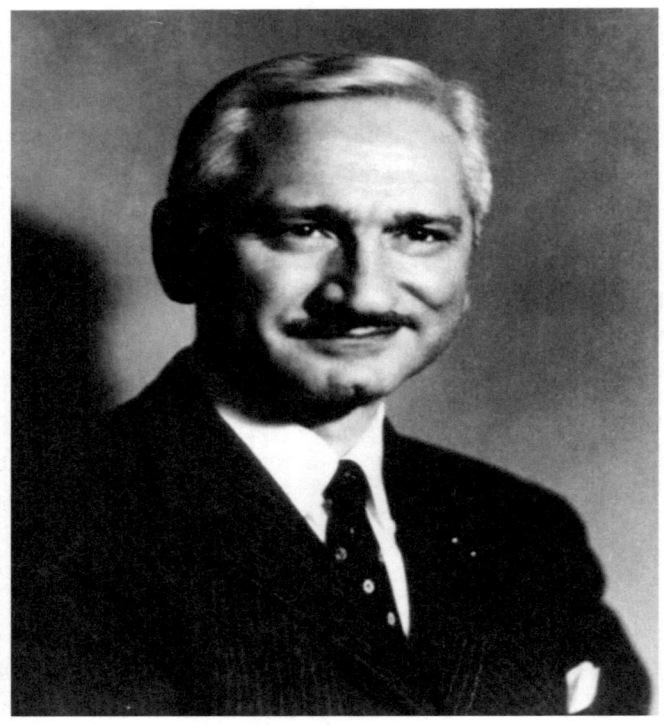

Albert Bruce Sabin, American Virologist

The previous year marked the death of 1,000 Jews in Odessa when 50,000 people roamed the streets of the city carrying pictures of Czar Nicholas 11 and shouting, "Down with the Jews." There were protests in the United States and 125,000 Jews marched in New York in sympathy with the plight of the Jews in the Russian Empire. His family immigrated to New York in 1921, the same year that British tanks started rolling over the cobbled streets of Dublin. Sabin was a good scholar and graduated from Pattison High School and went on to study dentistry. He felt bored with his course and entered the undergraduate program at New York University where he eventually received his MD degree in 1931. It was the same year that American lawmen began closing in on Chicago liquor baron, Al Capone. Sabin developed an interest in bacteriology while working with Professor W. H. Park, who encouraged him to take up research into polio. His MD thesis included research, which showed that the skin test used to determine polio was invalid. He first worked as a house physician at the Bellevue Hospital before going to the Lister Institute in London in 1933. He later returned to take up a position at the Rockefeller Institute a few years later. He moved to Cincinnati in 1939, at the start of the Second World War.

During the war, he served with the United States Army Medical Corps, during which he studied viral diseases threatening American troops in various parts of the world, including Japanese encephalitis, for which he developed a vaccine. Over the next thirty years, he worked at the University of Cincinnati College of Medicine and the Children's Hospital Research Foundation. In 1960, his oral polio vaccine was used in 100 million children in Europe. Between 1962 and 1964, 100 million persons of all ages received the vaccine in the United States. Estimates suggest that in just its first two years of worldwide use, the vaccine prevented half a million deaths and five million cases of paralytic polio.

****

In later years, Sabin investigated the relationship between viruses and cancer. He served as president of the Weizmann Institute of Sciences in Israel from 1970 to 1972, and in 1974, he joined the Medical University of South Carolina. He remained working there until 1982 when he moved to the Fogarty International Centre. Sabin continued to work into his eighties and had significant input into medical science and humanitarianism. When the definitive history of the 20th century is written, the achievements of Sabin will occupy a significant place.

Few in the history of science and medicine have contributed as much to the well-being of the world.

Sabin's most significant achievement was the development of the oral polio vaccine, which was an alternative to the inactivated polio vaccine developed by Jonas Salk. Sabin's vaccine utilized weakened forms of the poliovirus, providing immunity against the disease. He refused to patent his vaccine, waiving every commercial exploitation by pharmaceutical industries, so that the low price would guarantee a more extensive spread of the treatment. From the development of his vaccine, Sabin did not gain a penny and continued to live on his salary as a professor. Sabin's oral polio vaccine was easier to administer, more cost-effective, and provided long-lasting immunity. It played a crucial role in the global efforts to eliminate polio and has been instrumental in reducing polio cases worldwide. He conducted extensive research on viral diseases and made significant contributions to the fields of virology and immunology. He also made important discoveries related to other viruses, including viral hepatitis, dengue fever, and the Epstein-Barr virus. In addition to his work on vaccines, Sabin made significant contributions to the understanding of diseases such as toxoplasmosis and cancer. He conducted ground-breaking research on the relationship between viruses and cancer. Sabin's work earned him numerous accolades and recognition, including the Presidential Medal of Freedom, which he received in 1986. His contributions to public health and the eradication of polio have had a lasting impact on global health. Albert Bruce Sabin passed away on March 3, 1993.

I Am Flavivirus, Causer of Yellow Fever, and Who Held Up Construction of the Panama Canal.

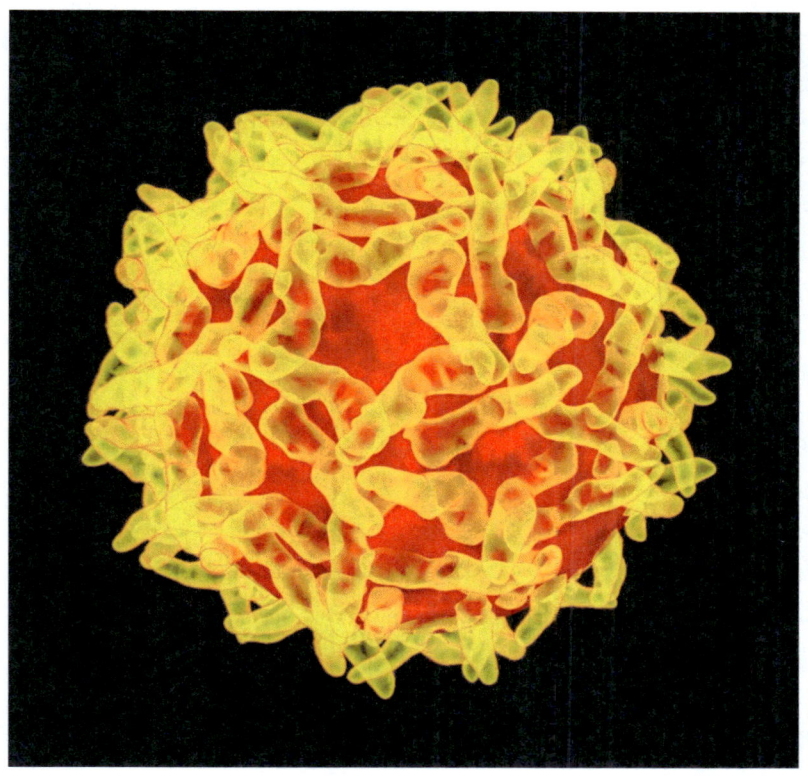

Yellow fever, an African mosquito-borne infection of primates has long been considered one of the most lethal and feared diseases. The disease is caused by a virus of the Flavivirus genus of the Flaviviridae family. Flavivirus is a genus of viruses that belongs to the Flaviviridae family. It includes several important human pathogens, such as yellow fever virus, dengue virus, Zika virus, and West

Nile virus. The Flavivirus genus is characterized by a single-stranded, positive-sense RNA genome enclosed in an envelope. These viruses are primarily transmitted by arthropods, particularly mosquitoes, although ticks also play a role in some cases.

Yellow fever virus (YFV) is one of the viruses within the Flavivirus genus. It is responsible for causing yellow fever, a viral disease primarily found in tropical and subtropical regions of Africa and South America. Yellow fever virus is transmitted to humans through the bite of infected mosquitoes, particularly Aedes aegypti and Haemagogus species mosquitoes. These mosquitoes acquire the virus by feeding on infected primates or humans. Yellow fever can cause a range of symptoms, including fever, headache, muscle pain, nausea, and jaundice (yellowing of the skin and eyes). Severe cases can result in organ failure, bleeding, and even death. It is one of those diseases that has jumped species, as in its natural habitat, it is transmitted between monkeys by Aedes mosquitoes. It infects only humans, other primates, and several types of mosquitoes. Most patients with yellow fever are asymptomatic, but among the 15% who develop severe illness, the case fatality rate is 20%–60%. Yellow fever is characterized by hepatic dysfunction, renal failure, coagulopathy, and shock. The midzone of the liver lobule is principally affected, with sparing of cells bordering the central vein and portal tracts.

In areas where yellow fever is endemic, the virus can be transmitted in a sylvatic (jungle) cycle involving non-human primates and forest-dwelling mosquitoes. However, it can also spill over into urban areas, leading to outbreaks. Vaccination is an effective preventive measure against yellow fever. The yellow fever vaccine, a live attenuated vaccine, provides long-lasting immunity against the virus and is recommended for individuals traveling to or living in areas at risk.

This is the story from the Yellow Fever virus's point of view.

I started my life in Africa and was carried to the Americas on ships during the slave trade era, by the ship of Spanish and Portuguese who were importing enslaved Africans from sub-Saharan Africa. Yellow Fever appeared in the U.S. in the late 17th century. My first memories of those journeys take me back nearly four hundred years, as I started spreading disease as early as 1648 in the Yucatan peninsula. It was the same year that England experienced its Second Civil War, and Oliver Cromwell's Parliamentarian troops defeated a Scottish-Royalist

Army. Soon I was on the march and started another epidemic in the bustling city of Philadelphia in 1699.

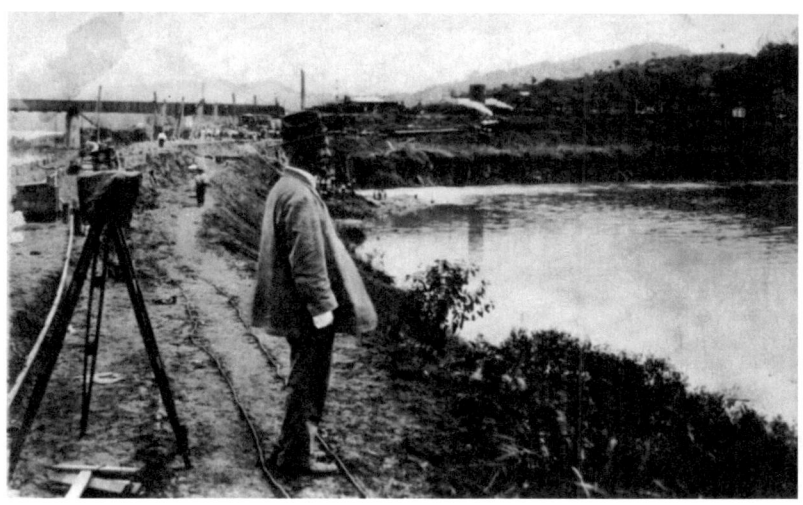

William C. Gorgas (1854–1920), on the site of Panama Canal construction

This was an interesting year, as down the coast a bit, investors from the Kingdom of Scotland attempted to gain the wealth and influence of their English neighbours by establishing a colony on the Isthmus of Panama, called New Caledonia. The plan was to establish and manage an overland route to connect the Pacific and Atlantic oceans. The scheme was backed by twenty percent of all the money circulating in Scotland, and its failure left the entire Lowlands in substantial financial ruin. This event changed history as it was an important factor in weakening their resistance to the Act of Union (completed in 1707). Both England and Spain opposed the colonial plan, afraid that Scotland would try and compete with them for territory. After just eight months, the colony was abandoned in July 1699, except for six men who were too weak to move but deaths continued on the ships, and only 300 of the 1200 settlers survived. It is amazing now to think that two hundred years after the turn of the twentieth century, the construction of the Panama Canal remained at a standstill. Needless to say, it was not because of a lack of political will or money, but rather because I had arrived and claimed the lives of thousands of new workers who tried to finish the Scottish job of constructing the canal. It seems that everyone was afraid to go to Panama because of 'Yellow Jack', the illness, which I caused, which resulted in high fever, vomiting, and even severe pain. Left untreated, it takes hold in the liver, resulting in jaundice that gives me my name. I continued to strike cities, mostly eastern seaports, and Gulf Coast cities, for the next two hundred years, killing hundreds, sometimes thousands in a single summer. Yellow fever broke out in Boston in 1693, Philadelphia in 1793 and Norfolk, Virginia in 1855, but the worst American outbreak of yellow fever occurred in the Mississippi River Valley in 1878.

By the 19th century, it was generally recognised that I was not a communicable disease and many theories existed until in 1881, Carlos Finlay of Cuba blew my cover and suggested that the *Culex cubensis* mosquito (now known as *Aedes aegypti*) was responsible for spreading the disease. Finlay was born on December 3, 1833, in Puerto Príncipe, Cuba, and passed away on August 20, 1915, in Havana, Cuba. Finlay conducted extensive research on me, trying to establish the transmission of yellow fever and proposed that the disease was spread by none other than myself…the Aedes aegypti mosquito! His research challenged the prevailing theory at the time that yellow fever was caused by filth or contaminated objects. In 1881, he presented his mosquito theory at the International Sanitary Conference held in Havana. However, thankfully for me, his ideas were initially met with scepticism, and it took several years for his work to gain acceptance. However, his research and findings laid the foundation for future studies on mosquito-borne diseases and ultimately led to the development of effective strategies for controlling and preventing yellow fever. To be fair, he was honoured with several awards and accolades for his discoveries. His contributions to the field of tropical medicine earned him recognition and praise, and today, Carlos Finlay is widely regarded as a pioneer in the field of tropical medicine and his research on yellow fever significantly contributed to our understanding of the disease.

During this same period, the United States invaded Cuba as part of its war with Spain. Hostilities started after an explosion occurred on the USS Maine in Havana Harbor, leading to U.S. intervention in the Cuban War of Independence. I must say that for every soldier who died in that battle, another thirteen passed away because of my services. The war ended in victory for the United States and signalled the end of the Spanish empire in the Caribbean and Pacific and gave the United States control over the former colonies of Puerto Rico, the Philippines, and Guam. In 1901, US physician Walter Reed was studying yellow fever just outside of Havana at the end of the conflict and confirmed the theory of the Cuban doctor Carlos Finlay that I was transmitted by a particular mosquito species, rather than by direct contact. It's hard to believe that doctors were only beginning to accept the germ theory of disease, especially as it had been proposed in the late Middle Ages by physicians including Ibn Sina in 1025. The Catholic Church suppressed a lot of medical knowledge that Islamic countries had gained from the original Greek school of Athenea, originally burning libraries and espousing the nonsense belief that everything is controlled by something in the heavens above and should not be tampered with. Of course, this gave them incredible control of the faithful as long as people remained ignorant. As you will read in this book, a transitional scientific period began in the late 1850s with the wonderful work of Louis Pasteur, and this was later extended by Robert Koch in the 1880s. Although there was no disputing the fact that Pasteur had shown quite convincingly that microbes not only existed but also caused disease, we must remember that this was only about fifteen years later, and many of the older doctors remained entrenched in their beliefs. One of the many proponents of this belief was a physician called Benjamin Rush, MD (1745–1813), who took it to exurbanite extreme to try and control me. He, like many other doctors, believed in another crazy theory that was left over from the days of Greek physician Hippocrates (460–370 BC) and] Galen (AD 129–c. 200). They believed there were four body humours: black bile, yellow bile, phlegm, and blood, and when you had an inflammation, they thought that if you removed blood, you would reduce the inflammation. Back then, humoral physiology was the key to medicine, and many believed that certain diseases and behaviours were caused by an excess or lack of body fluids, classified as blood, yellow bile, black bile, and phlegm. Medicine and science were kept in check with the Christian conquest of the bulk of the Islamic Iberian Peninsula took place in the 13th century. In 1492, the 'Catholic Monarchs', Ferdinand, and Isabella, took control of the last Muslim state in Spain, the emirate of Granada. They began with the reversal of freedoms beginning with the Alhambra Decree. Then Archbishop Talavera was replaced by the intolerant Cardinal Cisneros, who decided to have mass forced conversions and to publicly burn thousands of Arabic books with all the knowledge of thousands of years. In 1499, the Muslim leaders of Granada were ordered to hand over almost all of the remaining books in Arabic, most of which were burned. Many intellectuals tried to save the medical manuscripts, and some were put in safekeeping in the Escorial Library. However, the damage was done and when the Moorish doctors were treating their soldiers with surgery and plaster of Paris, the Christians were confined to trephination and bloodletting.

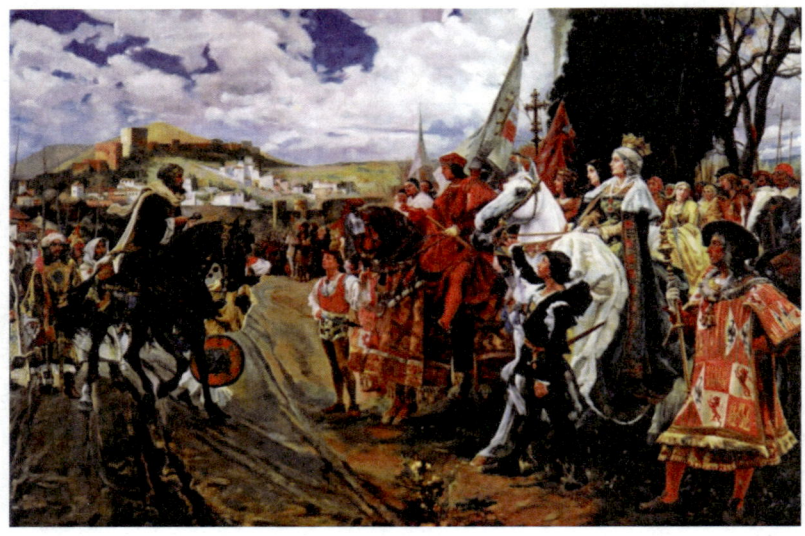

'The Capitulation of Granada'. Oil on canvas painting by Francisco Pradilla Ortiz (1848–1921)

In 1799, George Washington was about two-and-a-half years into his retirement and was still very actively managing his estate at Mount Vernon, Virginia. In the early morning hours of the 13th of December, following a day on horseback in freezing rain and snow, he woke up with pain from an inflamed throat. His aide-de-camp, Colonel Tobias Lear, sent out for some doctors and a bloodletter. After a series of medical procedures, including the draining of nearly 40 percent of his blood, by ten that night, he was dead. They also applied Spanish fly onto his throat, which raises a painful blister, again to remove these terrible humours that are causing the inflammation. In a nutshell, that's how bad medicine was.

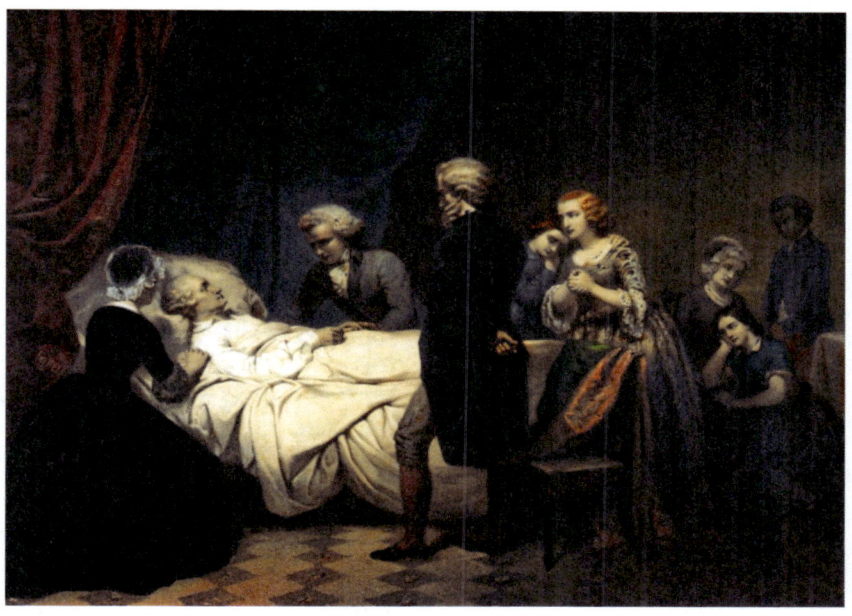

Print showing George Washington on his deathbed in 1799 surrounded by family and friends at his Mount Vernon plantation home.

However, to get back to Benjamin Rush, who later became one of the most well-known physicians in 18th century America, being also a philosopher, author, fervent evangelist, and politician. Rush graduated from an early Princeton University at age 14 and translated Hippocrates' Aphorisms from the Greek at age seventeen. He wrote the first textbook of chemistry to be published in America, one of the first of his eighty-five significant publications. In 1761, he decided on a career in medicine, and it is said Benjamin Franklin paid the costs of his education, as he wanted him for the position of professor of chemistry at the College of Philadelphia. He was by all accounts a devoted medical practitioner, who cared deeply for his patients' welfare, but his championship of extreme purging and bleeding created intense controversy, particularly illustrated by his behaviour during the Philadelphia yellow fever epidemic of 1793. Between August 1 and November 9, 1793, approximately 11,000 people contracted yellow fever in the US capital of Philadelphia. Of that number, 5,000 people, 10 percent of the city's population, died. The epidemic created panic in the capital, causing 17,000 people, including President Washington and other members of the federal government, to flee to the countryside. By excessive blood leeching and purging patients, Benjamin Rush decreased mortality but his controversial practices and unwillingness to listen to reason led to his resignation from the Philadelphia College of Physicians in that year. It is thought he removed so much blood from his patients that some got better as he actually reduced the viral load in the body.

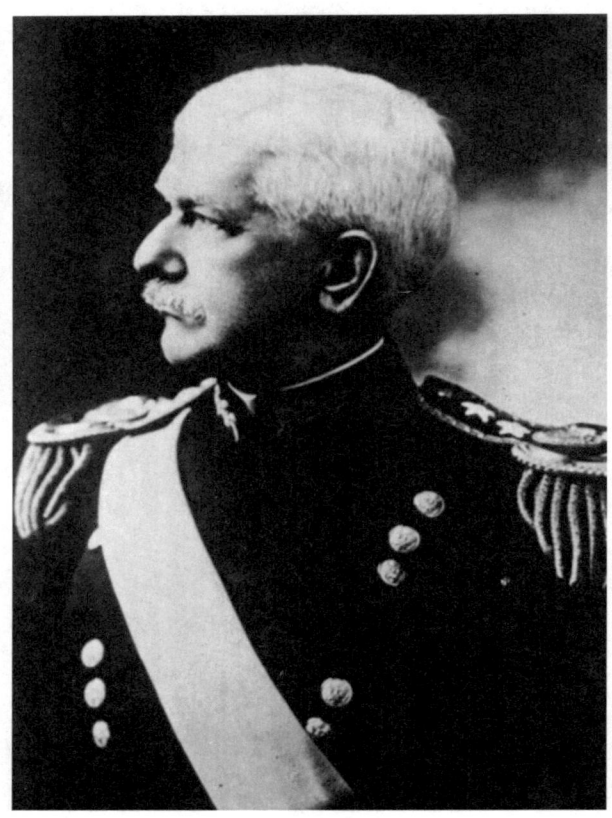

Major General William C Gorgas, United States Army physician who worked hard to combat Yellow Fever and Malaria in Panama, Havana, and Florida.

Meanwhile back at the Panama Canal, Major William C. Gorgas, previous Chief Sanitary Officer in Havana, Cuba, noted that Walter Reed had documented that Yellow Fever was transmitted by Aedes aegypti mosquitoes. He had instituted measures to destroy all Aedes aegypti breeding sites in Havana and within a few months, I had been eliminated from there and people started to look afresh at the Panama Canal Zone. True to form, Gorgas weeded me out by destroying Aedes aegypti breeding sites and finally, on November 11, 1906, the last victim of yellow fever on the Panama Canal died. The yellow fever epidemic was over, and this enabled the United States to resume construction of the Panama Canal, which was completed in 1914.

In 1927, the yellow fever virus was the first human virus to be isolated. Max Theiler, a South African-American virologist and physician, developed the first vaccine against me in 1937. He was awarded the Nobel Prize in Physiology or Medicine in 1951.

Yellow fever virus is estimated to cause 200,000 cases of disease and 30,000 deaths each year, with 90% occurring in Africa. 20% to 50% of infected persons who develop severe diseases die. There is no medicine to treat or cure the infection. To prevent getting sick from yellow fever, use insect repellent, wear long-sleeved shirts and long pants, and get vaccinated. After World War II, the world had DDT in its arsenal of mosquito control measures, and mosquito eradication became the primary method of controlling yellow fever. In 2013, yellow fever resulted in about 127,000 severe infections and 45,000 deaths worldwide, with nearly 90 percent of these occurring in African nations. Nearly a billion people live in an area of the world where the disease is common. The World Health Organization (WHO) states that a single dose of vaccine is sufficient to confer lifelong immunity against yellow fever disease.

I Am the Variola Virus, Which Caused Smallpox, Once One of the Greatest Scourges of Mankind

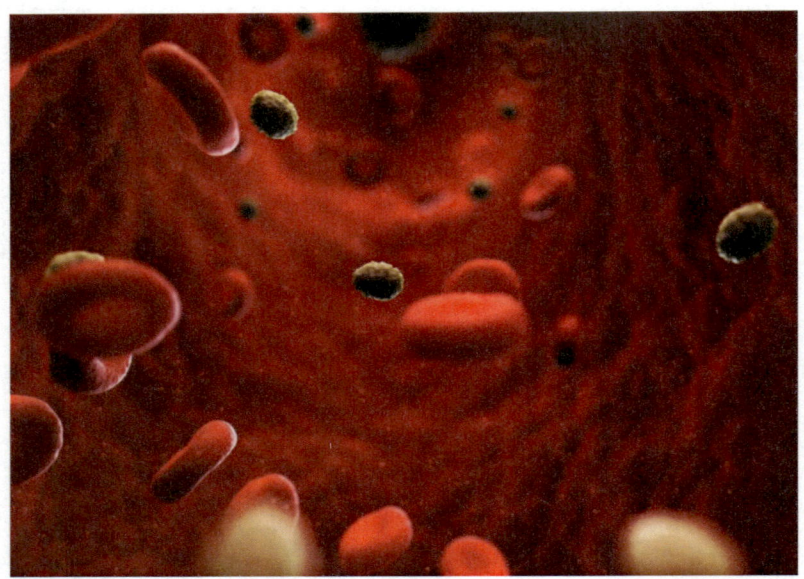

Introduction

Smallpox, a disease of antiquity, was one of the greatest scourges of mankind. In endemic form and in waves of epidemics, it killed and disfigured innumerable millions of people throughout the world. The Variola virus is the causative agent of smallpox. There are two types of Variola virus: Variola major and Variola minor. Variola major is associated with more severe symptoms and higher mortality rates, while Variola minor causes a milder form of the disease. Smallpox is transmitted from person to person through respiratory droplets. Close contact with an infected individual is required for transmission. The virus can also spread through direct contact with infected bodily fluids or contaminated objects. The symptoms of smallpox include high fever, fatigue, headache, and a characteristic rash that progresses from macules to papules, vesicles, and finally pustules. The pustules eventually scab over and leave permanent scars. Smallpox has a high mortality rate, especially in unvaccinated individuals. However, those who survive smallpox usually develop lifelong immunity.

During the 20th century, it is estimated that smallpox was responsible for 300–500 million deaths. Dr Edward Jenner introduced vaccination (using cowpox virus instead of smallpox virus) into Britain in 1796. As a result of widespread vaccination, smallpox declined steadily in Europe and North America. Elsewhere, however, death from smallpox prevailed. However, thanks to a global vaccination campaign, smallpox was declared eradicated in 1980, making it the first disease to be eradicated by human effort. In January 1967, The World Health Organization (WHO) initiated a program for the global eradication of smallpox. This was achieved in October 1977 when the last person to acquire naturally occurring smallpox in the world recovered from this disease in Somalia, Africa.

This is my story from the Variola virus's point of view.

I am the Variola virus, once one of the greatest scourges of mankind. I have been around for many thousands of years and descriptions of me appear in the earliest Egyptian, Indian, and Chinese writings. It is thought, I was there with Ramesses V, whose reign was characterized by the continued growth of the power of the priesthood of Amun. The circumstances of Ramesses V's death are unknown, but it is believed he had a reign of almost four full years but his mummy in the Cairo Museum suggests that he may have died from smallpox. We do know that he died at the age of forty in 1157 BC, but his mummified face still shows groups of pustules as well as others on his thorax and abdomen. In 1979, President Mohammad Anwar Al-Sadat allowed specimens to be collected for analysis and three other mummies in that period had similar lesions. We would have expected more cases if it was a pandemic. President Mohammad Anwar Al-Sadat served as the third President of Egypt, from 15 October 1970 until his assassination by fundamentalist army officers on 6 October 1981. Because everyone hated me, there are many ancient texts that show physicians attempts to eliminate my influence. A technique called *variolation* is found in the Sanskrit text 'Sacteya', and the Hindus even had a special God called Kakurani to deal with me. This willingness to religions to take advantage of people's lack of science and misery is seen time and time again across Hinduism, Christianity, and Islam and most of it involves paying money to some God to free a patient from their illness. François-Marie Arouet, known by his nom de plume Voltaire, the French historian, and philosopher famous for his criticism of Christianity, as well as his advocacy of separation of church and state, addresses this and mentions that the ancient Chinese inhaled dried powder of smallpox crusts through the nose as a means of halting me spreading. Persians were reported to have used a similar method Rhazes in 910 A.D. wrote about the difference between the symptoms between myself and my cousins in his classic monograph 'A Treatise on Smallpox and Measles', and he even stated that Galen knew about me in the second century. Abū Bakr Muhammad Zakariyyā Rāzī, was a Persian polymath, physician, alchemist, philosopher, and important figure in the history of medicine and I mention him in more detail in my book 'The Living History of Medicine' ISBN 9781398406490 (Paperback) ISBN 9781398406506 (EPub-e-Book). *www.austinmacauley.co.uk*

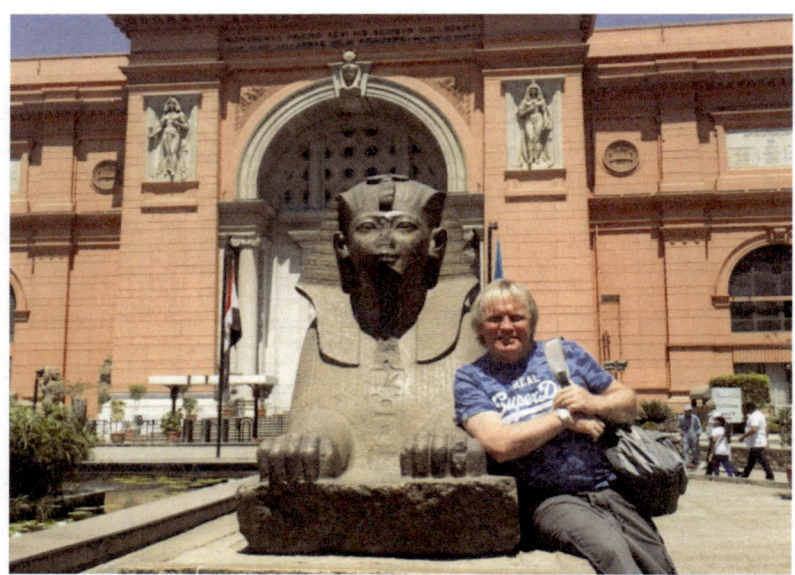

Author outside the Cairo Museum

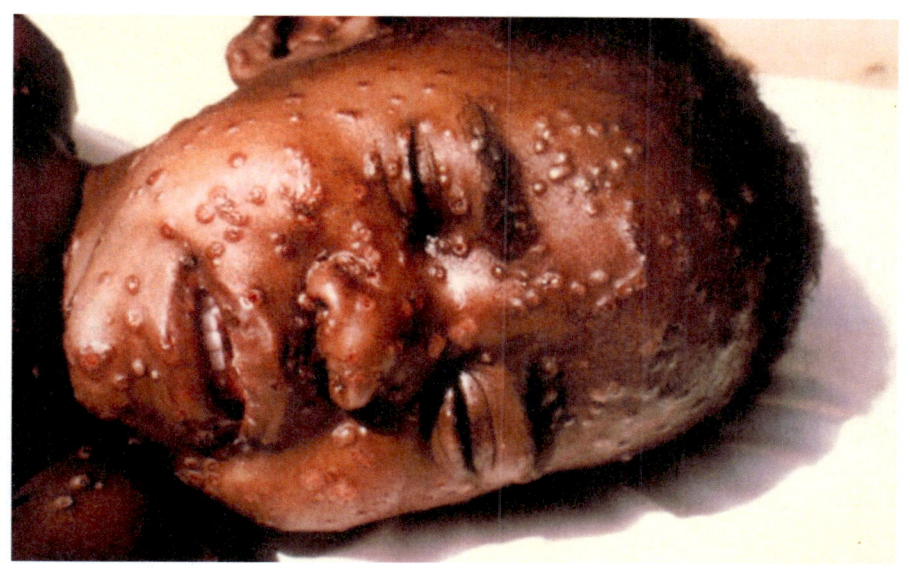

Smallpox patient with pustules

Variolation usually meant taking some of the pus from the pustules of a smallpox patient and using a stick to scratch it onto somebody's arm. This in itself was dangerous with the risk of giving a patient the whole disease rather than creating immunity by using a weakened version of the virus. The procedure was quite common in North Africa, Arabia, Turkey, and Greece, even though the people who did it know nothing about immunology or what they were doing. There is evidence that the Chinese were using the nasal route of variolation during the Sung dynasty (960 to 1280 A.D.). This period was considered the third Chinese golden age and divided almost evenly into Northern (960–1126) and Southern (1127–1279) halves. The former was a tranquil time characterized by philosophical and artistic development, political centralization, and economic growth. The latter, however, was quite the opposite; brutal invaders drove the Chinese from their northern territory, forcing them to migrate south and establish a new capital city. The psychological effects of this devastating upheaval are apparent in Sung's paintings of the period.

Thucydides, the Athenian historian and general (460–400 BC), who wrote about me in the history of the Peloponnesian Wars, and described an outbreak of smallpox that occurred in Athens around 430 B.C. He said that I hitched a ride aboard a ship coming from North Africa and docking at Piraeus (the port of Athens). Gregory of Tours in 580 A.D., also mentioned treating patients whom I had infected. The Koran mentions God sending flocks of birds to attack the Abyssinian army who were attacking Mecca to destroy the Kaaba, and them all ending up with sores and pustules that spread like a pestilence among the troops. The fact that the birds allegedly dropped stones on the vanquished army, means it was the first time I attacked a dive bomber. I was disseminated to North Africa and Europe during the sixth, seventh, and eighth centuries by the Arab invaders. Aaron of Alexandria, a contemporary of the Prophet Mohammad mentions that I was present in Cairo, Egypt around 570 A.D. It's amazing how wars can spread disease. Large concentrations of men, mostly undernourished, the lack of medical care, or any sanitation provide the vectors for illness to take hold.

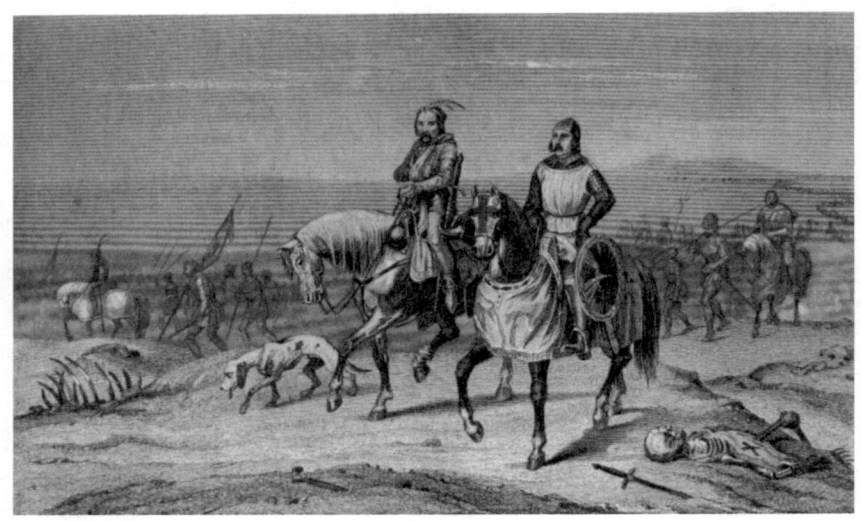

Return of the Crusader armies to Europe.

Even in the days before vaccination, the Crusader armies returning from wars in the Holy Land (1096 to 1291), carried me back to Europe. The syphilis pandemic of the 15th century was related to soldiers arriving back to France and Italy. About 5 years later, the Peruvian Empire, some 2,000 miles to the south, was devastated by smallpox. It is thought that the loss of so many people from this area directly affected climate change figures of the period.

It is believed that the Spanish Conquistador Hernando Cortes infected and killed some 3.5 million Aztec Indians during the smallpox epidemic of 1520 to

1522. In 1519, he left Cuba and was commissioned to lead an expedition to the shores of present-day Mexico, home of the Aztec Empire. When he landed, he ordered his small fleet of ships to be sunk so his 500 men were forced into the Mexican interior to the Aztec civilization, an empire of an estimated 16 million people. In 1520, another group of Spanish arrived in Mexico from Hispaniola, bringing me with them, as I had already been ravaging that island for two years. When Cortés heard about another group of Spanish arriving, he went and defeated them. During that conflict, I infected one of his men. Though vastly outnumbered, he and a small force marched on Tenochtitlan, where Montezuma received them with honour. In turn, Cortés took Montezuma prisoner and the Aztecs rose up in rebellion against him. Outnumbered, the Spanish were forced to flee.

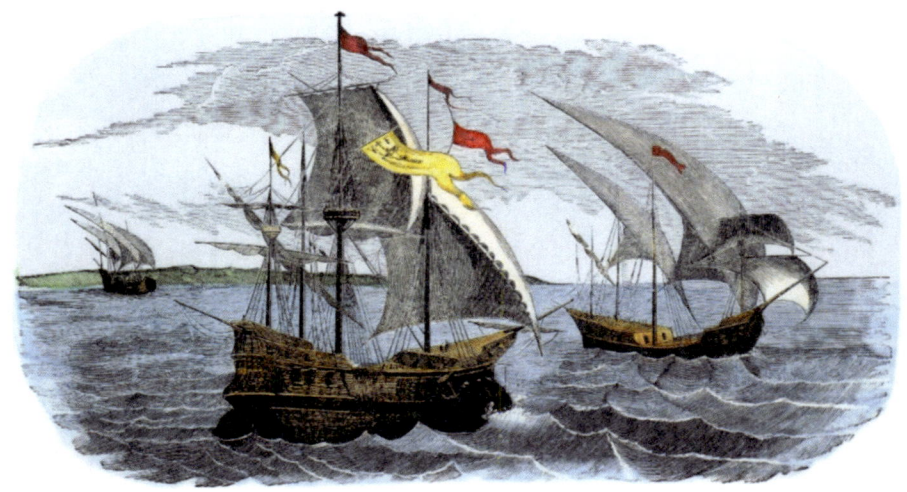

Spanish ships of Hernando Cortes sailing to Mexico 1519

In the meantime, my disease devastated the Aztec population, killing most of the Aztec army and 25% of the overall population. The next year, Cortés returned to Tenochtitlan and found the Aztec army in ruins. He then killed Montezuma and claimed the Aztec empire for Spain. There is little doubt that Cortés benefited from my assistance as I rapidly spread inward from the coast of Mexico and decimated the densely populated city of Tenochtitlan, reducing its population by 40 percent in 1520. Cortés was a skilled leader, but without my help, he, and his force of perhaps a thousand Spaniards and indigenous allies would not have been able to overcome a city of 200,000. The Spaniards said that they could not walk through the streets without stepping on the bodies of smallpox victims and the Franciscan monk Motolinia left this description: '*The Indians died in heaps, like bedbugs. In many places, it happened that everyone in a house died and, as it was impossible to bury the great number of dead, they pulled down the houses over them so that their homes become their tombs.*' The people could no longer tend to their crops, leading to widespread famine, and the destruction of their empire. The Aztecs were not the only indigenous people to suffer from the introduction of European diseases. In addition to North America's Native American populations, the Mayan and Incan civilizations were also nearly wiped out by smallpox.

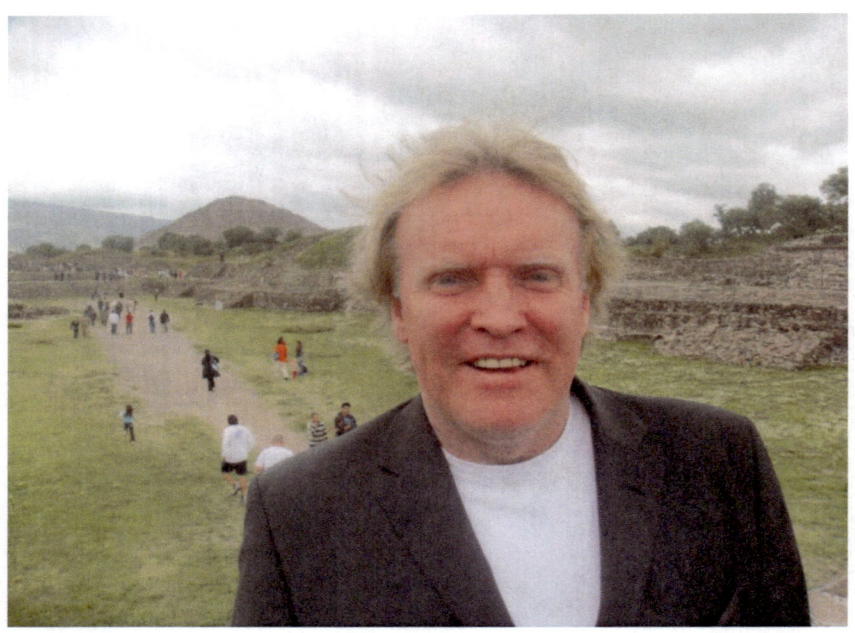

The author visiting Tenochtitlan

The differences were very noticeable during the Franco-Prussian War of 1870 to 1871. The French, who did not get vaccinated as protection lost 23,400 soldiers to smallpox, while the German army had only 278 dead from the disease. On 10th October 1562, twenty-nine-year-old Queen Elizabeth I was taken ill at Hampton Court Palace, with what was thought to be a bad cold. However, the cold developed into a violent fever, and it became clear that the young queen actually had smallpox. Just seven days later, it was feared that the Queen would die. She survived but it left her bald with permanent disfiguring facial scars. In 1694, Queen Mary II, who co-reigned with her husband, William of Orange over Ireland, Scotland, and England died from smallpox at age 32. It was not long after the Battle of the Boyne between the forces of the deposed King James II of England and Ireland, VII of Scotland, versus those of King William III who, with his wife Queen Mary II (his cousin and James's daughter), had acceded to the Crowns of England and Scotland in 1689. The battle took place across the River Boyne close to the town of Drogheda in the Kingdom of Ireland, the modern-day Republic of Ireland, and resulted in a victory for William. This turned the tide in James's failed attempt to regain the British crown and ultimately aided in ensuring the continued Protestant ascendancy in Ireland. The battle took place on 1 July 1690 O.S. William's forces defeated James's army, which consisted mostly of raw recruits. Although the Williamite War in Ireland continued until October 1691, James fled to France after the Boyne, never to return.

Introduction of Variolation into Britain

I mentioned earlier that the variolation type of immunization against smallpox was initiated hundreds of years ago in Asia and Africa. In China, India, Persia, and Africa. It was prominent in Turkey in the eighteenth century with documentation of the procedure being practiced in Constantinople in an earlier period. The physician and naturalist Patrick Russell (1727 to 1805) wrote in 1767 that variolation was commonly practiced by the Bedouins of the Middle East, including Iraq. Dr Russell was representative of the naturalistic tendency of British medicine in the late 18th century, being a keen observer and skilled doctor in clinical practice. His half-brother, Alexander and he recorded the life and times of people living through an outbreak of the plague, particularly in the Ottoman city of Aleppo, Syria. It is nearly two hundred years since the publication in 1796 of 'An Account of Indian Serpents collected on the Coast of Coromandel' and his study of plant and animal life both in Aleppo and later in the Madras Province of India, has left a rich legacy to this day. Smallpox was still a fatal disease throughout Western Europe, and because of Russel's data and a growing army of many reputable European physicians.

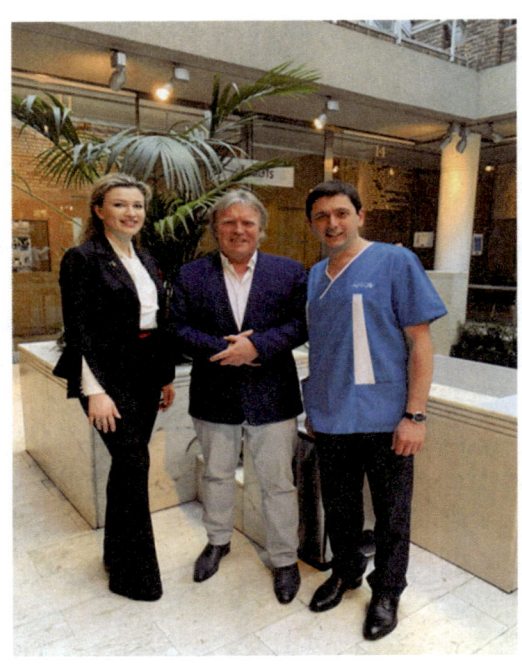

The author lecturing at the Royal Society London

The Royal Society of London became aware of variolation for protection against smallpox. They decided to investigate the process of variolation further and on the 14 February 1700, Dr Clopton Havers gave a lecture on the Chinese practice of the technique. He was able to reference reports from Joseph Lister, an East Indian Co. trader stationed in China, to Dr Martin Lister (1638 to 1712), already a member of the Royal Society. Later in 1712, Dr Edward Tarry of Enfield, who had returned to Britain from Pera and Galata, claimed to have observed more than 4,000 variolated persons. Moreover, the Scottish surgeon Dr Peter Kennedy described variolation in his book published in 1715. Because of Britain's prominence in foreign lands, through traders, ambassadors, and missionaries etc., the awareness of other nations' use of variolation as a means of controlling smallpox grew. Many important physicians said it was nonsense, and something practiced by Muslims. The Royal Society continued to investigate the possibility of the introduction of variolation into Britain. It gained the support of many prominent London physicians, including the Anglo-Irish physician, naturalist, and collector Sir Hans Sloane, who had been elected to the Royal Society at the age of 24. Sloane was a renowned medical doctor among the aristocracy and was elected to the Royal College of Physicians at age 27. As well as his collection of 71,000 items which the Ulsterman bequeathed to the British nation, he is credited with creating drinking chocolate. It is said that his collection provided the foundation of the British Museum, the British Library and the Natural History Museum, London. Because of recent protests against people involved with slavery, a bust of Sloane was removed in August 2020 from prominent display in the British Museum. Other doctors keen to see the use of variolation in Britain included and Dr James Jurin, Dr John Arbuthnot, Dr John Crawford, Dr Samuel Brady, Dr James Keith, and Dr Richard Mead, who after evaluating the collected statistical data, publicly endorsed the practice. It was at this stage, Lady Mary Wortley Montagu, the wife of Lord Edward Wortley Montagu, the British Ambassador to the Ottoman Empire, took a prominent role in the debate.

Lady Mary had a long history of involvement with smallpox. Like Queen Elizabeth 1, she had been stricken with smallpox in her twenties and had suffered deeply pockmarked skin and loss of eyelashes. Her brother had died of this disease, and while in Turkey, she became enthusiastically interested in the practice of variolation as a preventive measure against smallpox. In 1718, as the War of the Quadruple Alliance: Britain, the Kingdom of France, the Holy Roman Empire, and the Dutch Republic declared war on Spain, she variolated some of her children against smallpox, without her husband's knowledge. The Embassy Chaplain, was against the practice of variolation, stating that it was unchristian, and something practiced by Moslems. Her willingness to expose her children to the practice made many physicians take note and Dr Walter Harris, a physician to Queen Anne, mentioned it during a lecture given before the Royal College of Physicians on 17 April 1721. In 1749, Edward Jenner was born in Berkeley, Gloucestershire, in southwestern England. His father, the Reverend Stephen Jenner, was the vicar of Berkeley. In the summer of 1757, a smallpox epidemic broke out in Gloucestershire, and Jenner at the age of 8 years was variolated by an apothecary of Wooten-Under-Edge named Mr Holbrow. He suffered a lot of side effects, some of which remained throughout his life.

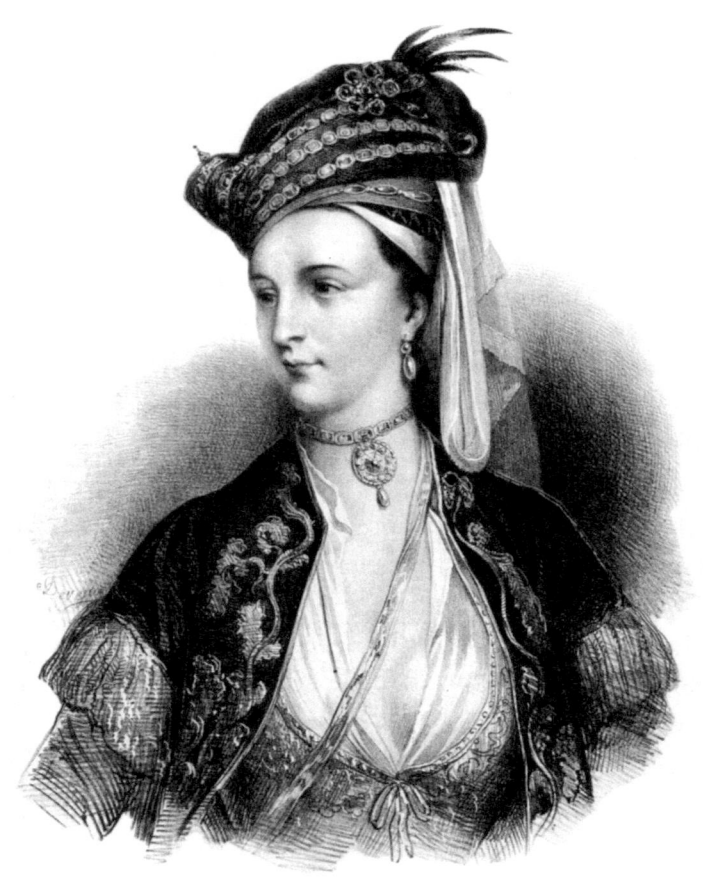

Lady Mary Wortley Montagu (1689–August 21, 1762) was an English aristocrat, letter writer and poet. Lady Mary is today chiefly remembered for her travels to the Ottoman Empire, as wife to the British ambassador to Turkey. The story of this voyage and of her observations of Eastern life is told in Letters from Turkey. During her visit, she was charmed by the beauty and hospitality of the Ottoman women she encountered.

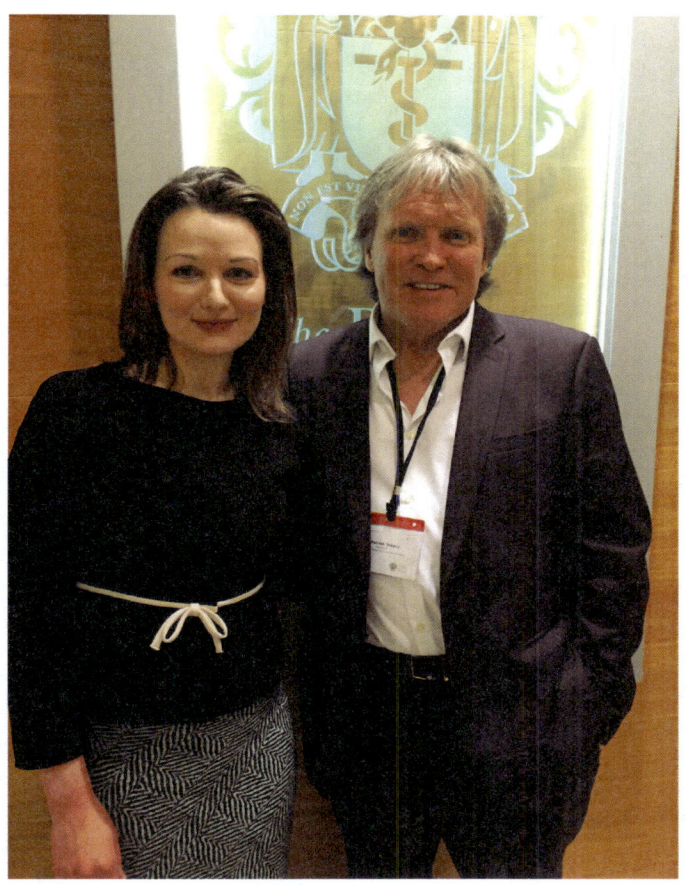

The author speaking at the Royal College of Physicians

By 1750, the practice of variolation gained some prominence in London, and physicians from other parts of Europe travelled to London to study the practice. Variolation was practiced in Holland, Switzerland, Sweden and Denmark in this period and Denmark in this period and publicly performed on two children in Paris in 1756 by Tronchin. There were similar public displays as with Covid vaccination today when the Duke de Chartres and Empress Maria Theresa publicly endorsed variolation.

In the winter of 1764, there was a smallpox epidemic in Boston and President John Adams went to get the variolation procedure against it. The President's cousin was a physician called Zabdiel Boylston, who became convinced of the benefit of the practice after speaking to a Puritan minister slave owner, Cotton

Mather whose slaves made him aware of the practice. Boylston began inoculating hundreds of Bostonians, but many physicians were against the practice and said that he was only spreading the disease. Boylston was physically assaulted on the street of Boston but recent data from Europe showed inoculation had dropped the smallpox mortality rate to 1% from approximately 15%. So many people became variolated and ignored the ban on its use, that in June 1776, Massachusetts suspended its prohibition, and many doctors set up shop in Boston to perform inoculations.

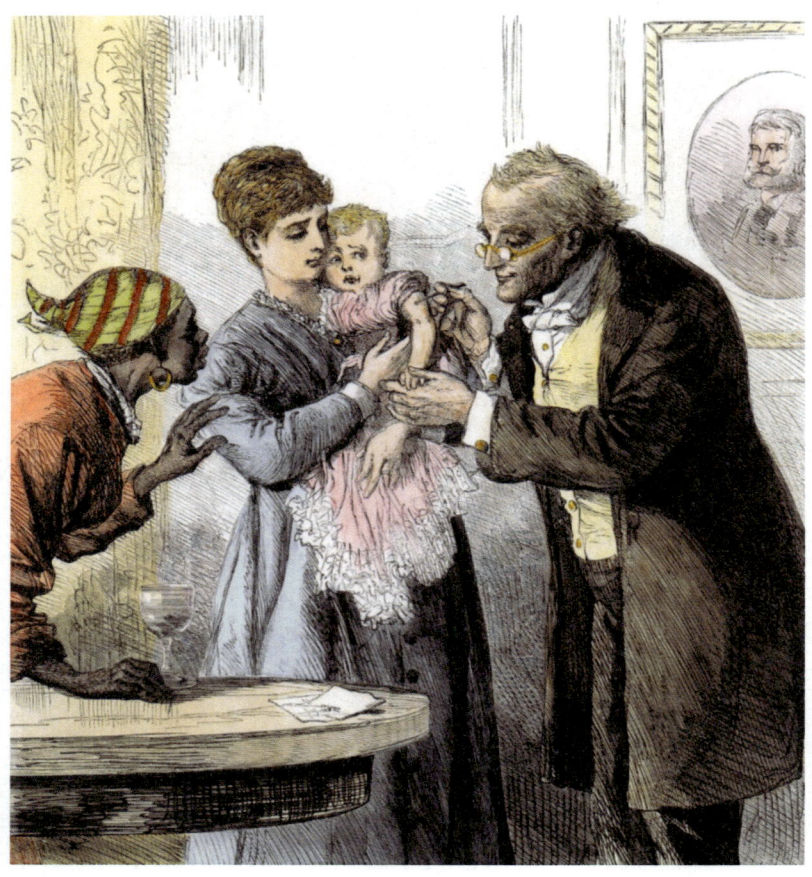

Physician vaccinating a baby against smallpox using live vaccine US circa 1870

In 1770, Jenner became apprenticed in surgery and anatomy under Dr Ludlow in Sodbury and surgeon John Hunter and others at St George's Hospital, London. While there, he had to treat some smallpox patients, and was informed by a dairymaid that the pustular skin infection that he was treating was cowpox, and the condition was well known amongst farmers in the area. In 1773, Jenner returned to Berkeley and became a successful family doctor and surgeon. He noted this in his 1801 book 'The Origin of the Vaccine Inoculation', and indicated that many of his patients who had contracted cowpox by milking cows with these lesions on their teats resisted variolation.

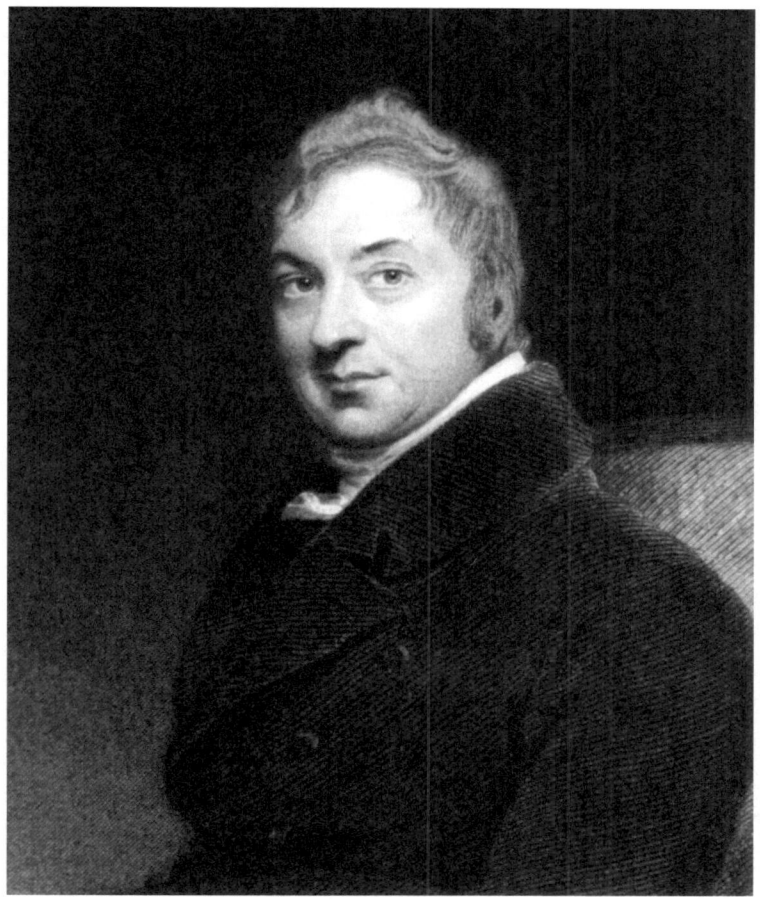

Edward Jenner, pioneer of smallpox vaccine, the world's first vaccine.

His other surgical mentor, John Hunter FRS was a Scottish surgeon, and one of the most distinguished scientists and surgeons of his day. He was an early advocate of careful observation and scientific method in medicine and learned anatomy by assisting his elder brother William at his anatomy school in Central London, starting in 1748, and quickly became an expert in anatomy. He is alleged to have paid for the stolen body of Charles Byrne, the Irish giant who was regarded as a curiosity in London in the 1780s due to his large eightfoot stature and proceeded to study and exhibit it against the deceased's explicit wishes. The remark about the protective effect of cowpox against smallpox remained with Jenner and he mentioned it to Hunter, who, as usual, suggested more experimentation and less speculation to prove the notion. It is said that Canadian physician and one of the four founding professors of Johns Hopkins Hospital, Sir William Osler, records that surgeon John Hunter gave Edward Jenner, William Harvey's advice, "Don't think about it; try it out." Osler has frequently been described as the *Father of Modern Medicine* and one of the "greatest diagnosticians ever to wield a stethoscope. It appears John Hunter remained in correspondence with Jenner over their combined interest in natural history and proposed him to become elected as a Fellow of the Royal Society."

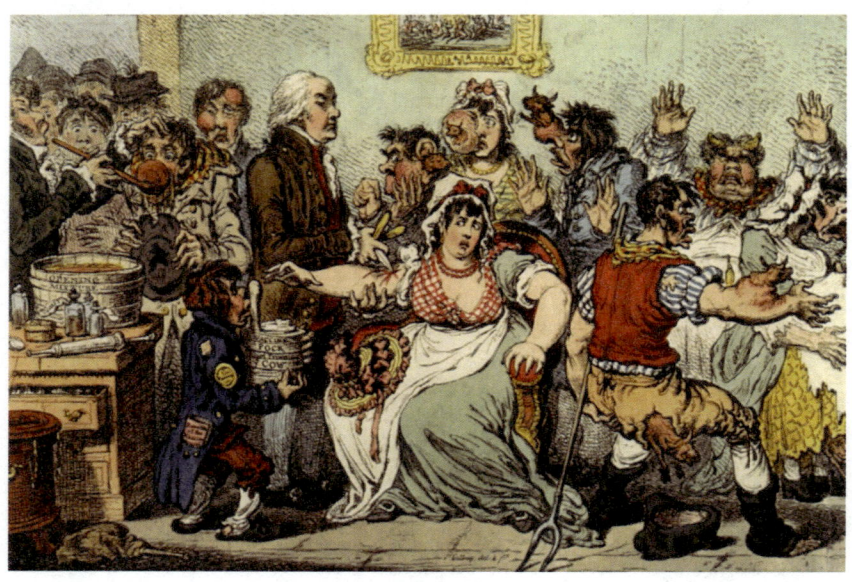

1802 cartoon shows Edward Jenner doing vaccinations at the Smallpox and Inoculation Hospital in St Pancras London the original caption proclaimed the treatment had Wonderful Effects and shows imaginary comic effects.

The opportunity came in 1788 after Jenner published a study of the nested cuckoo, in which he described how the newly hatched cuckoo pushed its host's eggs and fledgling chicks out of the nest (contrary to existing belief that the adult cuckoo did it). He even showed how the young cuckoos had adapted their anatomy by developing a depression in their back that enables them to cup eggs and other chicks. While in Berkeley, Jenner and some other doctors formed the Fleece Medical Society or Gloucestershire Medical Society, discussing topics of the day, including cardiovascular disease and cowpox. However, Jenner was not alone in considering the benefits of cowpox vaccination. It is well established that Benjamin Jesty, a cattle breeder from Dorsetshire vaccinated his family with material taken directly from the cowpox lesion of the udder of a cow. By 1768, English physician John Fewster had realised that prior infection with cowpox rendered a person immune to smallpox. Fewster was a surgeon and apothecary in Thornbury, Gloucestershire. Fewster, and a friend and professional colleague of Jenner. There is little doubt that he played an important role in the discovery of the smallpox vaccine. Many sources claim that in 1765, Fewster read a paper to the Medical Society of London titled 'Cowpox and its ability to prevent smallpox'. However, the Medical Society of London was created in 1773. In 1769, Jobst Bose in Germany pointed out the protection against smallpox acquired by milkmaids. However, this information was apparently not widely published until 1799. In 1781, it was reported that Nash wrote a paper on the natural history of cowpox, including its mode of spread in the herd through the milkers' hands and its protective effects against smallpox. There was another smallpox epidemic in 1778 that rekindled Jenner's interest in cowpox. Variolation was already a standard practice but involved serious risks, one of which was the fear that those inoculated would then transfer the disease to those around them due to their becoming carriers of the disease.

> AN
> # *INQUIRY*
> INTO
> ## THE CAUSES AND EFFECTS
> OF
> ## THE VARIOLÆ VACCINÆ,
> A DISEASE
> DISCOVERED IN SOME OF THE WESTERN COUNTIES OF ENGLAND,
> PARTICULARLY
> ## GLOUCESTERSHIRE,
> AND KNOWN BY THE NAME OF
> ## THE COW POX.
>
> BY EDWARD JENNER, M.D. F.R.S. &c.
>
> ———— QUID NOBIS CERTIUS IPSIS
> SENSIBUS ESSE POTEST, QUO VERA AC FALSA NOTEMUS.
> LUCRETIUS.
>
> London:
> PRINTED, FOR THE AUTHOR,
> BY SAMPSON LOW, N°. 7, BERWICK STREET, SOHO:
> AND SOLD BY LAW, AVE-MARIA LANE; AND MURRAY AND HIGHLEY, FLEET STREET.
>
> 1798.

1749–1823. Inquiry into the causes and effects of the variolae vaccinae.

As mentioned above, Jenner himself was variolated as a boy in 1756 and nearly died of the combined effects of the preparation and inoculated smallpox. Before his introduction of vaccination, Jenner practiced variation with increasing uneasiness and never showed any enthusiasm for it. Thus, the search for a safe and effective measure against smallpox was of immense importance to him. The terms *vaccine* and *vaccination* are derived from *Variolae vaccinae* (smallpox of the cow), the term devised by Jenner to denote cowpox. He used it in 1798 in the long title of his *Inquiry into the Variolae vaccinae known as the Cow Pox*, in which he described the protective effect of cowpox against smallpox. In the spring of 1763, a smallpox epidemic broke out near Fort Pitt, built by British forces between 1759 and 1761 during the French and Indian War at the confluence of the Monongahela and Allegheny rivers. A smallpox hospital was then also established there to treat sick troops. On June 24, of that year, William Trent, a fur trader, and merchant commissioned as a captain at the fort wrote a report in his journal about a meeting with two Delaware Indians at the fort. "*Out of our regard to them, we gave them two Blankets and Handkerchief out of the Smallpox Hospital. I hope it will have the desired effect.*" The two blankets and the handkerchief from the infirmary were unwashed and dirty.

In 1796, Jenner vaccinated James Phipps, the son of his gardener. He scraped pus from cowpox blisters on the hands of Sarah Nelmes, a milkmaid who had caught cowpox from a cow called Blossom, whose hide now hangs on the wall of the St George's Medical School library (now in Tooting). Phipps was the 17th case described in Jenner's first paper on vaccination, published in June 1798. He spent quite a bit of his own money producing a 64-page monograph with four coloured plates printed by Sampson Low of London. It was entitled '*An Inquiry into the Causes and Effects of the Variolae Vaccinae, a Disease Discovered in Some of the Western Counties of England Particularly Gloucestershire and Known by the Name of 'Cowpox'*. Jenner dedicated the work to his friend Dr Caleb H. Parry of Bath. Determined to disseminate information about the beneficial effects of vaccination, Jenner published three more books: '*Further Observations on the Variolae Vaccinae*' (1799), '*A Continuation of Facts and Observations Relative to Variolae Vaccinae or Cowpox*' (1800), and '*The Origin of the Vaccine Inoculation*' (1801). The second edition of An Inquiry with added data and a dedication to the King was presented to His Majesty by Jenner in person on 7 March 1800. After the introduction of vaccination in 1796 by Dr Edward Jenner, the incidence of smallpox declined steadily in Europe and North America. Like the proposed introduction of a Covid 19 vaccine passport today, smallpox vaccination became legally compulsory in many European countries, and soon the infection became of lesser importance as a cause of death among children than measles and scarlet fever. Smallpox, however, continued to be a great scourge among the Europeans even decades after the introduction of the Jennerian vaccination, and was present in most of the major cities of Europe during the eighteenth century. It is estimated that the disease killed 400,000 people each year and caused more than one-third of all the blindness in Europe at the end of the eighteenth century. It no respecter of class differences, and five European reigning monarchs (Joseph I of Germany, Peter II of Russia, Louis XV of France, William II of Orange, and the last Elector of Bavaria) succumbed to this disease during the eighteenth century.

In 1851, Francis Parkman was the first historian to document Lord Amherst's 'shameful plan' to exterminate Indians by giving them smallpox infected blankets taken from the corpses of British soldiers at Fort Pitt in 1763. Smallpox was used as a biological weapon during the French and Indian Wars (1754–1767) by the commander of Fort Pitt. Soldiers distributed blankets that had been used by smallpox patients with the intent of initiating outbreaks among American Indians. An epidemic occurred, killing more than 50% of infected tribes.

Letter by Edward Jenner regarding vaccines.

During the 1770s, smallpox killed at least 30% of the North-western Native Americans, killing tens of thousands. The smallpox epidemic of 1780–1782 brought devastation and drastic depopulation among the Plains Indians. By 1785, the Sioux Indians of the great plains had also been affected. William Walker in the 'Cumberland House Journals and Inland Journals 1775–82', described the epidemic stating that "the Indians are all dying by this distemper, lying dead about the barren ground like rotten sheep, their tents left standing and the wild beasts devouring them."

Smallpox reached Australia in 1789 but didn't reach New Zealand until April 1913, when the disease was introduced to Auckland by a Mormon missionary from Utah. Then, as now New Zealand used its benefit of being an island to try and protect themselves against the illness. In 1798, an insurrection was launched by the United Irishmen, who aimed at overthrowing the Kingdom of Ireland and severing the connection with Great Britain to establish the Irish Republic based on the principles of the French Revolution. In that year, Jenner went to London with a supply of his vaccine and tried in vain, to convince his colleagues of the validity of his immunization procedure.

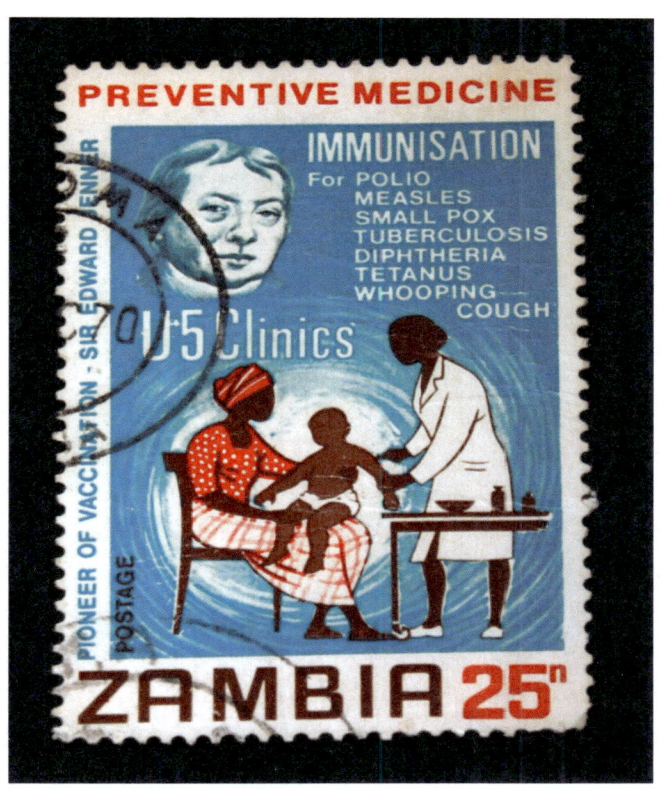

Postage stamp commemorating Edward Jenner

However, his vaccine was ridiculed by his colleagues as unnatural and dangerous. He was subjected to abuse in lectures and on the street and confronted with cartoons showing vaccinated babies growing cow-horns or cows erupting from inoculation sites. In 1805, they tried to humiliate him as a fraud and invited the old farmer, Benjamin Jesty, and his son Robert to London as inventors of the vaccination procedure. Most interesting of all was a letter of thanks sent to him in 1807 by the chiefs of the Five Nations of the North American Indians. The letter said: "Brother, our father has delivered to us the book you sent to instruct us how to use the discovery which the Great Spirit made to you whereby the smallpox that fatal enemy of our tribe may be driven from the earth. We send with this a belt and a string of wampum in token of our acceptance of your precious gift." When you consider the hundreds of thousands of native Americans deliberately killed by the use of contaminated blankets in the United States, this letter is difficult to turn away from. Jenner was appointed Physician Extraordinary to His Majesty King George IV on 16 March 1821, two years before his death. He was buried in the vault of Berkeley Church beside his beloved wife Catherine on 3 February 1823.

The medical establishment deliberated for over twenty years over his findings before accepting them. Many physicians in positions of authority, openly called Jenner a charlatan. Eventually, vaccination was accepted, and in 1840, the British government banned variolation – the use of smallpox to induce immunity – and provided vaccination using cowpox free of charge. In 1881, Louis Pasteur adopted the term vaccination for his newly developed anthrax vaccine, as a tribute to Jenner. As technology improved, the cowpox vaccine virus was obtained from bovine lymph and mixed with glycerol to improve storage. We can see today how important this is, as we analyse the differences and benefits of using an Astra Zeneca, Pfizer or Moderna vaccine. In the end, Jenner received many honours and awards from emperors and kings and from various groups and organizations throughout the world. Napoleon, who was at war with Britain, released English prisoners of war at Jenner's request, stating that he could not refuse such a humanitarian. Thomas Jefferson, the philosopher, and Founding father who served as the third president of the United States praised him for erasing 'from the calendar of human afflictions one of its greatest'.

In 1947, the worldwide incidence of smallpox between 1924 and 1947 was published by the World Health Organisation the number of countries where smallpox occurred had decreased from 79 to 69 but variola minor continued to occur in Canada and the United States, but the number of cases became much fewer. As we all watch as scientists develop new vaccines for the Covid 19 coronavirus, it's important to remember the controversies surrounding smallpox vaccination and that during the developments and adoption of vaccines, it is common to have initial disagreements among experts on treatments and often the first workable treatment is later replaced with an improved option.

I Am the Ebolavirus, Which Caused Haemorrhagic Fever and Instilled Fear into the Heart of Africa

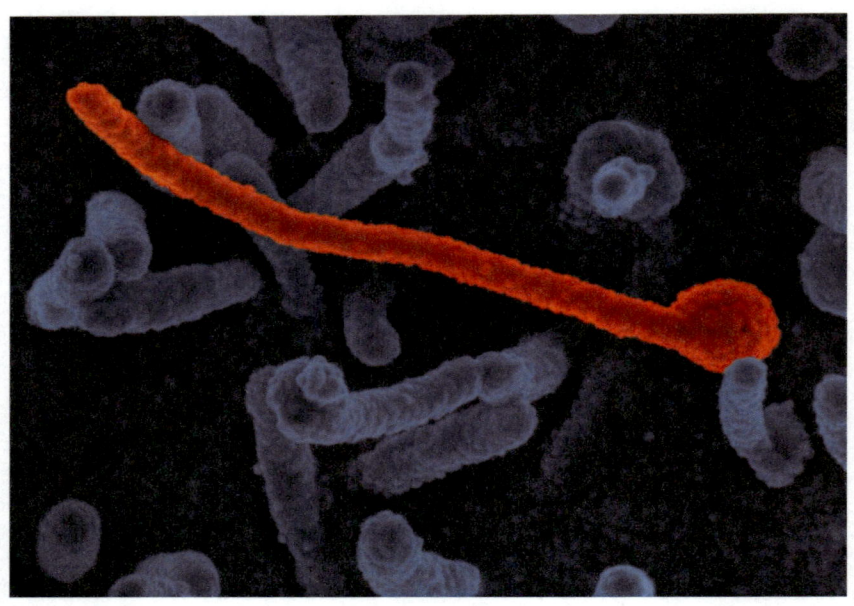

Ebola virus disease (EVD), commonly known as Ebola, is a severe and often fatal illness caused by the Ebolavirus. It belongs to a genus of viruses belonging to the family Filoviridae. There are five species of Ebolavirus: Zaire ebolavirus (EBOV), Sudan ebolavirus (SUDV), Taï Forest ebolavirus (TAFV), Bundibugyo ebolavirus (BDBV), and Reston ebolavirus (RESTV). Among these, EBOV is the most well-known and associated with severe outbreaks. The disease is primarily transmitted to humans through direct contact with the blood, secretions, organs, or other bodily fluids of infected animals such as fruit bats, chimpanzees, gorillas, monkeys, forest antelope, and porcupines. Human-to-human transmission occurs through direct contact with the blood, secretions, organs,

or contaminated surfaces of infected individuals. The symptoms of Ebola typically appear between two to 21 days after infection. They include sudden onset of fever, fatigue, muscle pain, headache, sore throat, and impaired kidney and liver function. As the disease progresses, it can lead to severe internal and external bleeding.

Ebola outbreaks have occurred primarily in Central and West African countries. The largest Ebola outbreak in history occurred in West Africa between 2014 and 2016, resulting in thousands of deaths. However, smaller outbreaks continue to occur sporadically. Diagnosis of Ebola involves laboratory testing of blood or other body fluids. Early detection and prompt isolation of infected individuals are crucial for preventing the spread of the virus. There is currently no specific treatment for Ebola, but supportive care such as fluid replacement, maintaining electrolyte balance, and treating other infections can improve survival rates. Experimental treatments and vaccines have shown promise in recent years. The Ebola vaccine is an important tool in preventing the spread of Ebola virus disease. The first licensed vaccine for Ebola is called ERVEBO (Ebola Zaire vaccine). It is a replication-competent, live, attenuated recombinant vesicular stomatitis virus (rVSV) vaccine manufactured by Merck. The vaccine contains a modified form of the vesicular stomatitis virus that expresses a protein from the Zaire ebolavirus.

ERVEBO was approved by the U.S. Food and Drug Administration (FDA) in December 2019. It is used for active immunization against Ebola virus disease caused by Zaire ebolavirus in individuals 18 years of age and older. The vaccine has been shown to be highly effective in preventing Ebola virus disease. It has been used in outbreak response settings and to vaccinate individuals at high risk of exposure, such as healthcare workers and frontline responders. The vaccine is administered as a single-dose injection. It stimulates an immune response in the body, which provides protection against Ebola if a vaccinated person is exposed to the virus. In addition to ERVEBO, there are other experimental Ebola vaccines and vaccine candidates being researched and developed. These include other recombinant vesicular stomatitis virus-based vaccines and viral vector-based vaccines. Vaccination alone is not sufficient to control Ebola outbreaks. It is important to implement comprehensive outbreak response measures, such as surveillance, contact tracing, isolation, and safe burial practices, in conjunction with vaccination.

Picture above: A scanning electron micrograph of Ebola virus Makona (in red) from the West African epidemic shown on the surface of Vero cells (blue). Early during the recent Ebola epidemic in West Africa, scientists speculated that the genetic diversity of the circulating Makona strain of virus (EBOV-Makona) would result in more severe disease and more transmissibility than prior strains. However, using two different animal models, National Institutes of Health scientists have determined that certain mutations stabilized early during the epidemic and did not alter Ebola disease presentation or outcome.

This is the story from the Ebola virus point of view.

I Am Ebolavirus, responsible for haemorrhagic fever, in both humans and primates and one of the most feared diseases on the planet. In fact, I have five brothers, responsible for many African diseases, Ebola virus (EBOV), Sudan virus (SUDV), Reston virus (RESTV), Taï Foi rest virus (TAFV), and Bundibugyo virus (BDBV). As you can see, I travel widely creating panic wherever I go. We are often carried from place to place by three different fruit bats, and consequently do them no harm. I got my unusual name from a river in in the northern Democratic Republic of the Congo, where I first came to light in a man from a small village called Yambuku in 1976. The fact the Ngbandi locals call the river, Legbala, meaning 'white water' and Ebola is a Belgian French corruption of the name (*L'Ébola*) is not really of my concern. For those who are interested, the village is about seven hundred miles northeast of Kinshasa, which we mentioned earlier in this novel, just so you know where we are. Yambuku could only be reached via government planes and helicopters, and communication with the outside world was all but impossible.

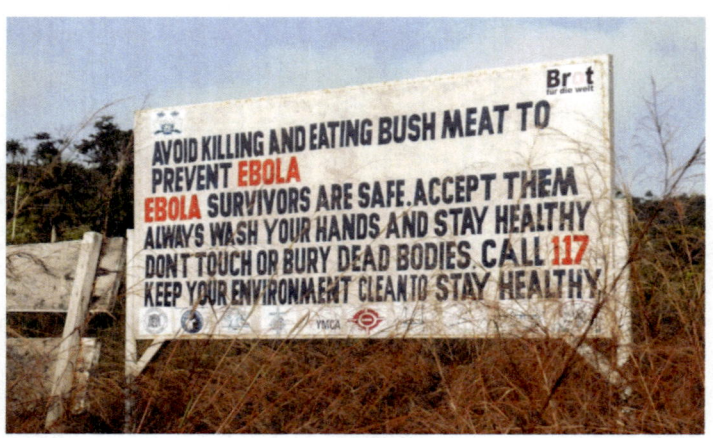

Above all people, he was the village schoolmaster, and his name was Mabalo Lokela, who had been well until he returned from a trip to Northern Zaire near the border of the Central African Republic, where he visited the now famous Ebola River. His local doctor thought he had developed malaria and prescribed him some quinine. As his symptoms worsened, he was admitted to Yambuku Mission Hospital where he died a few weeks later. His symptoms began a bit like malaria beginning with an influenza-like syndrome, including fever, headache, and joint and muscle pains, but when the schoolmaster a rash and haemorrhagic problems, his doctors knew something different was causing the problem. After the schoolmaster died, many other with whom he had been in contact also died. When one in two people who got the disease became ill and died, people in Yambuku began to panic and Zaire's Minister of Health and declared the entire region, including the country's capital, Kinshasa, a quarantine zone. But even though no-one was permitted to enter or leave the area, and all roads, waterways, and airfields were placed under martial law, my brother began a similar panic in Nzara, a small village in South Sudan, a landlocked country in East-Central Africa. I know those still awake will say that no such country existed back in 1976, and you are correct as it did not receive its independence until 2011, but anyway to confuse you even more, is bordered to the east by Ethiopia, to the north by Sudan, to the west by the Central African Republic, to the southwest by the Democratic Republic of the Congo, to the south by Uganda and to the southeast by Kenya. And you thought finding Kinshasa was difficult.

My brother infected nearly three hundred people and killed about fifty percent of them, between June and November 1976, starting with a storekeeper at a cotton factory in Nzara and later spreading to spread to the nearby villagers of Maridi and Juba. The storekeeper developed haemorrhagic problems on the fifth day of illness with profuse bleeding from the nose and mouth, and bloody diarrhoea. He was admitted to hospital in Nzara on 30 June and a week later. He was nursed by his brother, who became ill but survived. Another storekeeper who worked with him also died. As more people began to die, the Government of the Democratic Republic of Sudan asked the World Health Organisation to investigate the cause of my illness. This team worked closely with their Sudanese colleagues and with staff provided by other governments, identifying the virological and serological investigations. Two strains of a virus were isolated from acutely ill patients in Maridi hospital and antibodies to this virus were detected by immunofluorescence in nearly all the forty-eight patients there but less in Nzara. The team checked blood samples from the local community and discovered that nearly twenty percent had antibodies, despite not having any symptoms of the illness. One in three of the workers in the Nzara cotton factory virus had antibodies, suggesting this virus was probably the prime source of infection. The disease in Maridi was apparently amplified by transmission in that hospital and may have been spread by the nurses who were in close contact with the dying patients. They also established the incubation period of the illness was between 7 and 14 days. Although the link was not well established, it appears that my brother could Have been the source of infection for a similar outbreak in the Bumba Zone of Zaire.

Anyway, back to the first person that I infected with the disease, headmaster Mabalo Lokela, who began displaying symptoms on 26 August 1976. To deal with this outbreak, the World Health Organisation sent another team of Congolese doctors, led by microbiologist Jean-Jacques Muyembe-Tamfum. Jean-Jacques, presently General Director of the Democratic Republic of the Congo *Institut National pour la Recherche Biomedicale* (*INRB*). At the start of the outbreak, Muyembe-Tamfum was studying in Europe when he was called by his government regarding a mysterious disease killing people at the Catholic mission in Yambuku in Equator province. In truth, he was the country's only virologist at that time. The small international team of virus hunters who gathered in Zaire's capital, Kinshasa, knew little about the strange disease except for its horrible toll. They travelled overland by jeep to reach the mission hospital deep in the heart of the Equatorial forest. There was nobody in the hospital when they arrived, and the team decided to bed down in the mission for the night. Overnight, three nurses had died as well as some people in the village and the hospital was overflowing with patients. They entered villages to find entire families sprawled inside dirt-floored huts, crying out in hallucinations, moaning in pain, and bleeding from every orifice—blood that was filled with contagious viruses. Believe it or not, even though Muvembe drew blood from all these patients, he never got infected by me and lived to tell the tale.

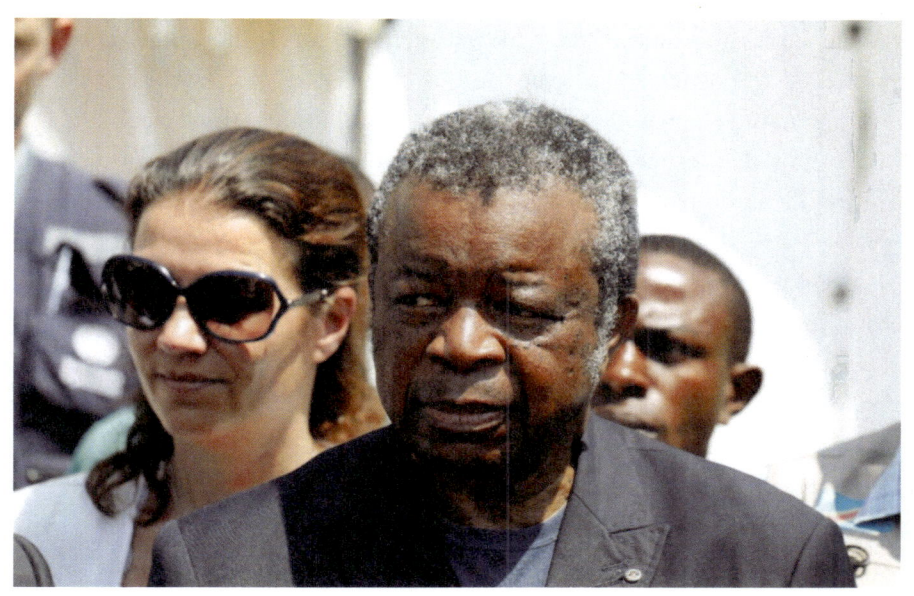

Congolese government's Ebola response coordinator Jean-Jacques Muvembe visits the new MSF (Doctors Without Borders) Ebola treatment centre in Goma, in the Democratic Republic of Congo Alamy Stock Photo

He even went further and took samples from the dead, from which I was still highly infective. It is said that he never even wore gloves during these procedures. Worse still, many of these patients kept bleeding because one of my special features was to stop blood from clotting. When some of the Belgium nuns started to become ill, he persuaded her to travel back with me to Kinshasa. Not knowing how deadly I was with close contacts they all shared jeeps, cars, and planes to make the arduous journey. Her blood samples were sent from Kinshasa to Belgium where scientists thought she had the Marburg virus, which was causing haemorrhagic fever in Uganda and the Congo. The patients all had symptoms that closely resembled the features described in this illness and their blood showed focal eosinophilic necrosis in the liver and destruction of lymphocytes and their replacement by plasma cells. One case even had evidence of a similar renal tubular necrosis.

Within a short period, all of the Belgian nun's travelling companions started to die and Muvembe realised how reckless he had been regarding his personal protection and he locked himself up in his garage, refusing to meet any of his family or friends. Meanwhile in Belgium, microbiologist Peter Piot identified me from the nun's blood as the cause of the mysterious African illness and named my virus after the Ebola River. Piot became director of the London School of Hygiene and Tropical Medicine and a pioneering researcher into AIDS. Muvembe never received any credit except becoming the first scientist to come in contact with me and survive. Interestingly, I have never been shown to transmit the virus from human to human through the air, although this may happen in primates. It is known that bushmeat, which is widely used in these parts provides an opportunity for transmission of several zoonotic viruses from animal hosts to humans, such as Ebolavirus and HIV. The spread of Ebola by water, or food other than bushmeat, has not been observed. No spread by mosquitos or other insects has been reported.

During Christmas 1994, I re-emerged in Zaire in the town of Kikwit, the largest city of Kwilu Province on the Kwilu River in the southwestern part of the Democratic Republic of the Congo. A local called Gaspard Menga was out in a nearby forest trying to find wood that he could burn down to charcoal and sell as fuel. It appears he came in contact with me through some animal while camping there. While nobody really knows how I spread from animals to humans, let me tell you the chances are it involves some type of contact with an infected wild animal or fruit bat. Maybe he ate bushmeat that he had hunted, although this was apparently denied. This type of food remains a primary source of animal for inhabitants of humid tropical forest regions in Africa, Latin America, and Asia, and remains an important food resource for poor people, particularly in rural areas. I also infect several species of monkeys such as baboons, great apes (chimpanzees and gorillas), and a species of antelope. Pigs can also spread me by coughing or sneezing causing droplets in the air. Either way, Menga brought me back with his firewood to the densely populated town of Kikwit and within a few days, not only was he was dead but had spread me to all the nearby villages.

The town of Kikwit was backward even by African standards with no effective clean water or sanitation and soon the populous was burying the dead in mass graves. It is known that basic medical facilities were manned by a few medical students and Doctors Without Borders, an international humanitarian medical non-governmental organisation which was started by a small group of French doctors, including a friend of mine, Yves Illouz to expand medical care across national boundaries and irrespective of race, religion, creed, or political affiliation, they heroically stopped me in my tracks within three months. Médecins Sans Frontières was founded in 1971, just after the Republic of Biafra, attempted to gain independence from the rest of Nigeria. This caused the Nigerian Civil War of 1967 to 1970 and a number of French doctors volunteered with the French Red Cross to work in hospitals and feeding centres in besieged Biafra. Only the Catholic countries of France, Spain, Portugal, and Ireland supported Biafra, while the United Kingdom, the Soviet Union and the United States sided with the Nigerian government.

By 2013, the world had witnessed twenty Ebola epidemics in Africa, but the worst was yet to come. In that year, I created havoc in Western Africa by creating the world's worst Ebola epidemic that lasted three, causing major loss of life and disrupted the economies of Guinea, Liberia, and Sierra Leone. The first cases were recorded in Guinea in December 2013; soon I spread to neighbouring Liberia and Sierra Leone.

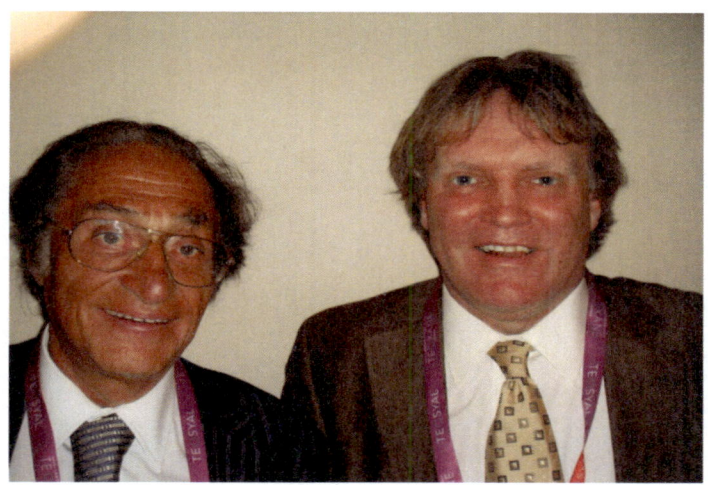

The author with Yves-Gérard Illouz (1929–2015) French surgeon, co-founder of Médecins Sans Frontières (Doctors Without Borders).

That Christmas, I created havoc in Western Africa by creating the world's worst Ebola epidemic, which lasted three more years, causing major loss of life and disrupting the already tattered economies of Guinea, Liberia, and Sierra Leone. The first cases were recorded in Guinea in December 2013; and soon I spread disease to the neighbouring nations of Liberia and Sierra Leone. By June 2014, the West African outbreak was the largest in Ebola's history spreading to cities with international airports, and overwhelmed the ability of Médecins Sans Frontières, or local government clinics and hospitals to deal with it. Before the outbreak of the Ebola epidemic, Liberia had only fifty doctors for a population of 4.5 million, and the country's health system was devastated after a civil war just a decade before. Many of the infections were caused by burial with infected corpses, especially in Guinea and Liberia, where nothing had been learned from previous burial rituals noted in Yambuku nearly forty years before. Dead bodies remain infectious; any person handling the dead remains was totally at risk of contracting the disease. In August 2014, the Liberian government ordered all corpses of those who died to be cremated.

On March 15th 2015, a 44-year-old woman from the Caldwell district of Monrovia destroyed any hope That Liberia, (one of the three West African countries hit by the Ebola epidemic that had killed more than 10,000 people since it began a year before), would be declared free of the virus.

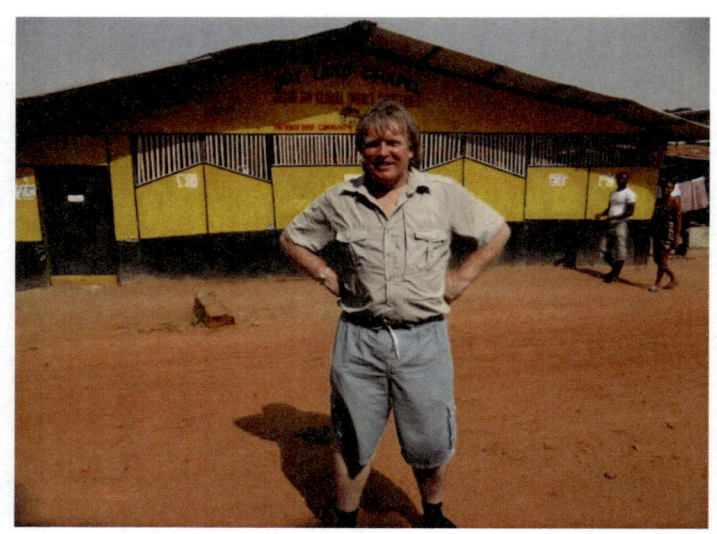

The author in Caldwell, Monrovia at the start of the 2014–2016 Ebola outbreak in Liberia

In response, UNICEF responded by deploying 20 additional general community health volunteers to the hotspot and neighbouring communities. As suspected cases of the Ebola virus continued to rise in Monrovia, another suspected victim, Dr William M. Tandapolie of the Caldwell community, died that June 25, as a result of contracting the disease, sources said. The world started to take notice as it was predicted that Liberia and Sierra Leone would have one million Ebola cases by February 2015, and that the two countries could lose up to 14 percent of their populations, as the epidemic continued.

In 2014, four laboratory-confirmed cases of Ebola occurred in the United States. Thomas Eric Duncan, a traveller from Liberia was diagnosed with the illness in Dallas, Texas, eight days after his arrival in the U.S., and he died a few days later. Some of the nurses who attended him at the Texas Health Presbyterian Hospital in Dallas caught the disease but survived. In December 2014, Pauline Cafferkey, a Scottish aid worker, who had been working at an Ebola treatment centre in Kerry Town in Sierra Leone was diagnosed with Ebola at Gartnavel General Hospital in Glasgow. She was transferred to the Royal Free Hospital in London and underwent intensive medical treatment, before being released from the hospital free of infection.

In 2016, J. J. Muyembe-Tamfum led the research that designed, along with other researchers from the Institut National pour la Recherche Biomedicale (INRB) in the Democratic Republic of Congo and the National Institute of Health Vaccine Research Center in the US, one of the most promising treatments for Ebola, mAb114. The drug, *Ansuvimab*, sold under the brand name Ebanga, is composed of a single monoclonal antibody (mAb) and was isolated from the blood of a survivor of the 1995 outbreak of Ebola virus disease in Kikwit, Democratic Republic of Congo roughly ten years later. The treatment was successfully used in the Democratic Republic of Congo, despite advice from the World Health Organization. Nigeria was the first country in western Africa to successfully curtail the virus, and its procedures have served as a model for other countries to follow. In December 2016, a study found the VSV-EBOV vaccine to be 70–100% effective against the Ebola virus, making it the first proven vaccine against the disease. In December 2019, the first vaccine to be approved in the United States was rVSV-ZEBOV. It had been trialled in the Kivu Ebola epidemic under an emergency approval. It was developed by the Public Health Agency of Canada, and later produced by Merck Inc.

****

A condition called post-Ebola syndrome has been noted in patients who have recovered from infection with Ebola. This has been noted in many other people who survived viral illness and symptoms include joint and muscle pain, eye problems, including blindness. Like Covid 19, other patients develop various neurological problems, sometimes so severe that the person is unable to work.

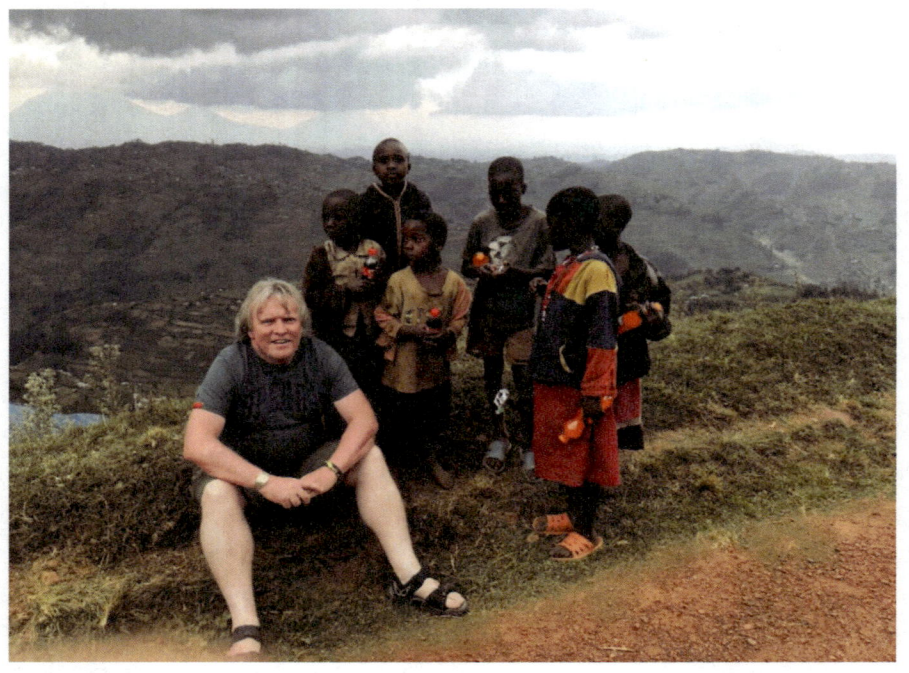

The author in the Virunga Hills Uganda at the end of the 2023 Ebola outbreak

The last outbreak of Ebola in Uganda was caused by the Sudan ebolavirus. The outbreak occurred in Uganda and was caused by the Sudan ebolavirus, one of the species of Ebola virus. Sudan ebolavirus is named after the country where it was first identified. The outbreak was declared over on January 11, 2023. The declaration was made by the Ugandan authorities after the successful containment of the outbreak. The affected areas during the outbreak included districts such as Masaka, Mubende, and Wakiso in Uganda. The World Health Organization (WHO) and other international health organizations collaborated with the Ugandan government to respond to the outbreak. This involved implementing measures such as case identification, contact tracing, isolation, treatment, and community engagement. The successful containment of the outbreak highlights the effectiveness of coordinated efforts in controlling Ebola outbreaks and preventing further spread of the disease.

I Am the Human Immunodeficiency Virus, Who Caused Worldwide Panic Before They Tamed Me

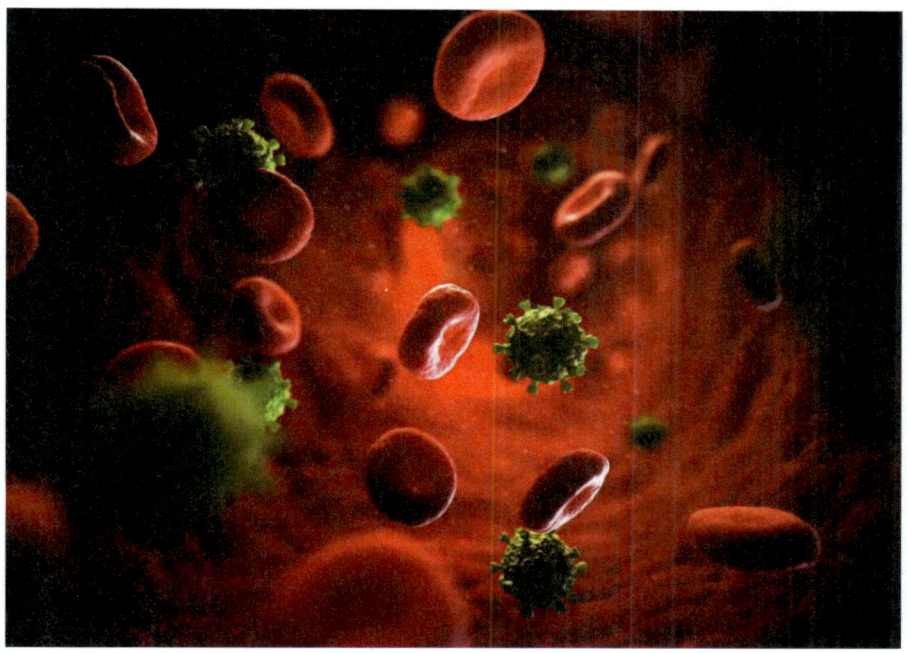

HIV (human immunodeficiency virus) is a virus that attacks the body's immune system. If HIV is not treated, it can lead to AIDS (acquired immunodeficiency syndrome). There is currently no effective cure. Once people get HIV, they have it for life.

I am the Human Immunodeficiency Virus and I have been on the planet for quite a lot longer than most people suspect. Many people think that I started my life the United States of America during the 1980s when Phil Collins was charting with 'Something In The Air Tonight', but truth be told I was already living in the town of Kinshasa in the Democratic Republic of Congo when Elvis Presley was singing with The Jordanaires and charting with 'A Big Hunk o' Love'. In fact, I was there forty years earlier but living in…a lowly chimpanzee. How did that happen? Well, at the risk of boring you, I am a lentivirus. We are slow viruses, playing the long game with incubation periods of months, or even years. We also can cause a wide range of diseases in many animal species. According to the most recent classification from no less a body than the International Committee on Taxonomy of Viruses (ICTV), we belong to the family Retroviridae and currently comprise of nine species: seven animal lentiviruses and two human lentiviruses. Sounds more Roman than the Democratic Republic of Congo but what can we do? Our first claim to fame was back in 1843, from the observation of the equine infectious anaemia in France. The young Queen Victoria had assumed the throne and Britain claimed the former Boer republic of Natal as a British colony.

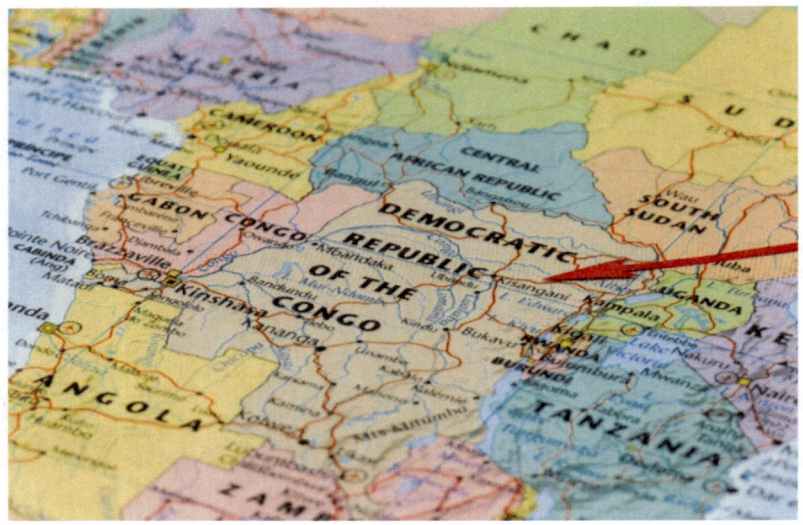

The origins of the HIV pandemic were in Kinshasa

I know you are thinking how did I cross from chimps to humans? Well, the most commonly accepted theory is that of the 'hunter' as a result of chimps being killed and eaten, or their blood getting into cuts or wounds on people in the course of hunting. Normally, humans would have this fought off, but on a few occasions the virus adapted itself within its new human host and became HIV-1.

My family caused a stir in the 1950s, when some sheep in Iceland got infected with a slowly progressive disorder in sheep was noted in Iceland during the 1950s caused by visna/maedi virus (VMV), which represented a severe form of pneumo-encephalopathy. In the 1960s, American researchers determined we also caused both leukaemia and lymphosarcoma in cattle, and the causative factor was a retrovirus bovine immunodeficiency virus (BIV), a cousin morphologically similar to VMV.

Anyway, enough of the science, did I tell you what a virus is? Let's start at the beginning. Life itself is divided into six kingdoms – animals, plants, bacteria, archaea (bacteria-like organisms living in extreme conditions), protists (e.g., amoebae) and fungi. The fundamental unit of each lifeform is the cell. Every cell is surrounded by a fatty membrane and can grow and divide into two daughter cells. We unfortunately are not included in the six kingdoms of life because we are not cells. The scientists feel we are not actually alive, but just hijacking living host cells to replicate ourselves. We have three families, spherical, rod-shaped, and mixed. We cause diseases in humans, including common colds, influenza and chickenpox, and more serious diseases like smallpox, Ebola and Covid 19.

Viruses, like myself, are small parasites with either an RNA or DNA genome that are surrounded by a protective protein coat and transfer our genetic material to infected cells. In other words, we have stripped down all of the elements of life to the most basic. Consider this as a staff member, going into a Chinese factory late at night to make extra iPhones. They have the knowledge to assemble the components but without the key to the factory door, they cannot survive. We are nothing more than a single iPhone motherboard wrapped in a plastic case. Many say: because we cannot survive without the key to the door, we are not really alive, but I really beg to differ. There is currently no consensus regarding the definition of life. Some say the definition should only be applied to organisms that are composed of cells, have a life cycle, undergo metabolism, can grow, adapt to their environment, respond to stimuli, reproduce, and evolve. Well, we're still here after many millennia and reproducing away. It is true, we have stripped back so much we only have a small number of genes. My cousin who causes Covid 19 only has about fifteen genes, as opposed to the twenty-five thousand genes found in a human being. Not having the complete personal protective package (cell membrane) leaves us vulnerable to hostile attack, and it is well known a little bit of soap or alcohol in a hand sanitiser is enough to completely disable us. President Trump unfortunately explained this phenomenon when he suggested injecting human with disinfectant.

Yes, we do lack the machinery to read DNA, to make proteins, or even to carry out metabolic processes. So, technically we can do nothing in isolation, especially the ability to reproduce. However, once we get inside the factory (cell), we quickly shed our disguise (protein envelope) and release nucleic acids into the cell. Our genetic code, (like the staff member) hijacks the machinery of the cell, giving it the message to produce more iPhones (viral progeny). In this way, the virus transforms living cells into virus-producing factories. Unfortunately, by analogy, the staff member overworks the machines he is using, and in the process the viruses destroy the host cells they have invaded. The newly formed mature viral particles then exit the host cells and move on to attack and invade new cells. As we make more copies of ourselves, we tend to destroy more and more cells, and the effect on the body can be severe or even catastrophic. The outcome is really dependent on the level of factory security, and whether the immune system contains or destroys the invasion. Enough said, let's move on.

Where was I? Down in Kinshasa. Now let me tell you about this town. You might never have heard of it but let me assure you it is a breeding ground of virus experimentation. Kinshasa is Africa's third-largest urban area after Cairo and Lagos. The area around Kinshasa is full of transport links, such as roads, railways, and rivers, and it is from here that I ventured to nearby Brazzaville in 1937. Scientists now have DNA evidence from histology samples that I visited there, when Count Basie, Bing Crosby, Fred Astaire, and Duke Ellington, were around. That particular year, Ella Fitzgerald was in the charts with 'Goodnight, My Love'.

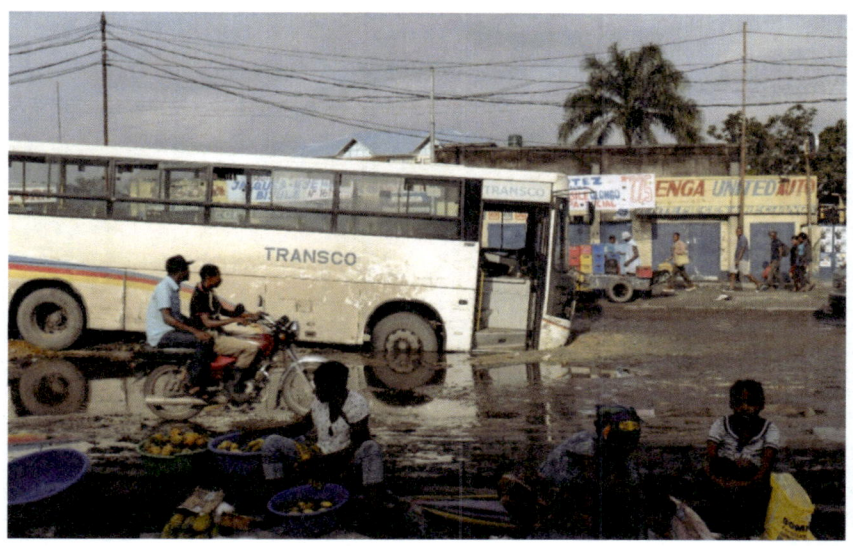

Kinshasa, Democratic Republic of the Congo. This is how the streets look after a rainfall in the rainy season. A bus is stuck in the mud, and shops and people's homes are flooded with water.

Kinshasa is also the world's largest Francophone urban area, with French being the language of government, schools, newspapers, public services, while Lingala is used as a lingua franca in the street. The area also had a growing sex trade around the time, and I used this as a means of spreading further along the truck routes where these people tend to assemble. Today, it's only a five-minute flight from Kinshasa to Brazzaville, but back then we had to cross an international border, the Congo River and centuries of colonialism left it easier to travel by boat. The lack of transport routes into the north and east of the country meant that it took me longer to spread in to these areas. Anyway, there were quite a lot of Haitian teachers working in the colonial Democratic Republic of Congo during the 1960s and I hitched a ride with one of them all the way back to Haiti.

By 1981, I had spread around the rest of the Democratic Republic of the Congo and started appearing in American a few cases of rare diseases were being reported among gay men in New York and California, such as Kaposi's Sarcoma (a rare cancer) and a lung infection called PCP. Kim Carnes was in the charts with 'Bette Davis Eyes' and John Lennon was singing '(Just Like) Starting Over'. Nobody really knew why these cancers and opportunistic infections were spreading, but doctors rightly concluded that there must be an infectious 'disease' causing them. I was beginning my journey into the United States and before long, had created enough panic that they began to close airports to prevent the rest of my family arriving. In 1983, some researchers at the Pasteur Institute in France identified me. They called me the Lymphadenopathy-Associated Virus (or LAV) and scientists working at the USA National Cancer Institute isolated my son called it HTLV-III. The game was up when LAV and HTLV-III were later acknowledged to be the same virus and confirmed as the cause of AIDS.

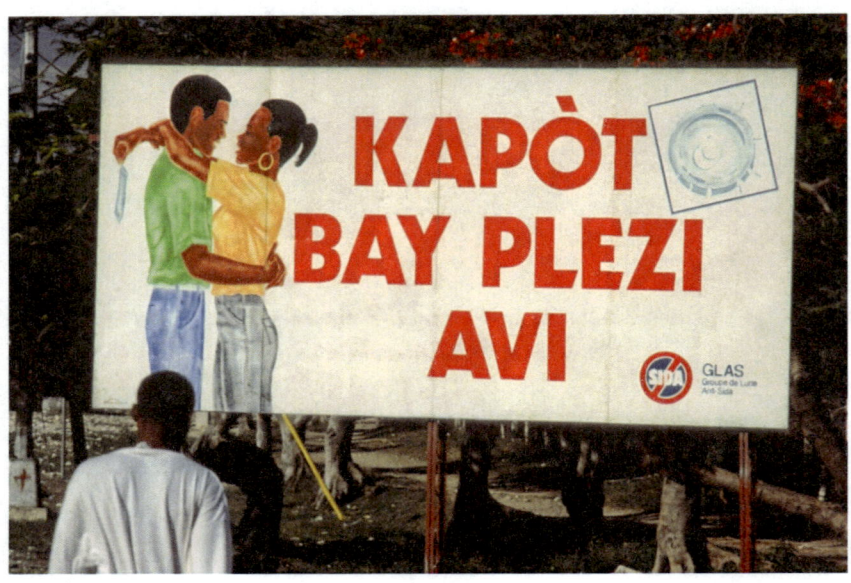

Mural encouraging use of condoms to prevent HIV Aids, in the streets of Port au Prince Haiti

Haiti still has the highest overall cases of HIV/AIDS in the Caribbean with over 150,000 people infected. Like South Africa, there are many risk factors groups for HIV infection there, with the most common ones including lower socioeconomic status, lower educational levels, risky behaviour, and low levels of public awareness regarding how HIV is transmitted. Levels are improving as educational campaigns begin to show some effect. A lot of controversy still remains about whether HIV was spread into the US by Haitians or vice versa. The controversy began in the 1982, when it was noted that over thirty cases of immunodeficient patients were Haitian. In the same period, we had the term 'the

4-H's' referring to Homosexuals, Haemophiliacs, Heroin addicts, and Haitians as the major groups prone to HIV infection.

By the end of the year 1981, I was on the march across the United States, where there were now nearly 300 cases of AIDS among gay men, and over one hundred had died. By next June, as Paul McCartney and Stevie Wonder released Ebony and Ivory, it was quite obvious that I was using sexual contact as a means of transmission and doctors in.

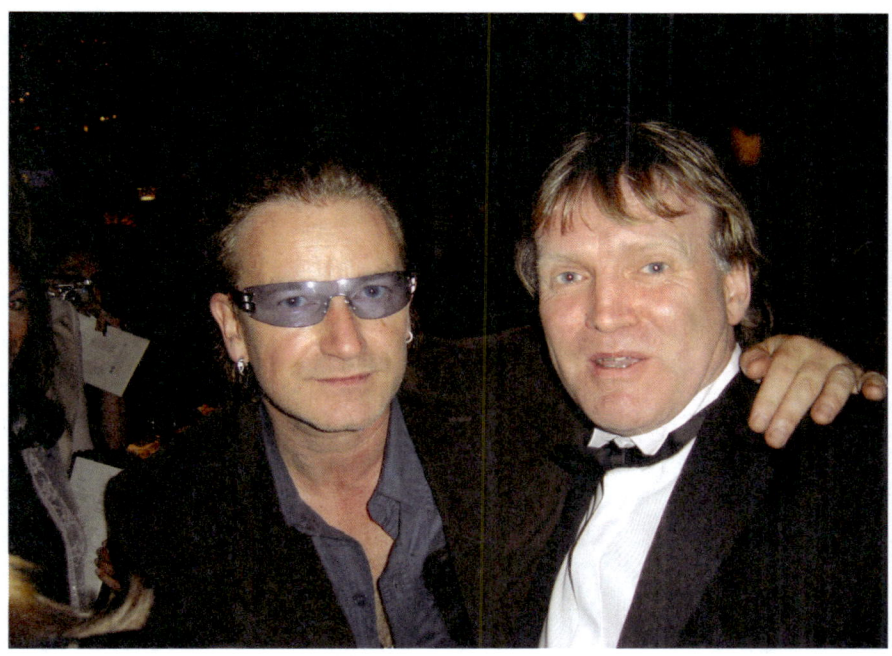

At the UN Millennium HIV/AIDS Goals New York (2003)

Los Angeles suggested the disease should be called gay-related immune deficiency (or GRID). Around this time, my good friend, the late Arnold Klein wrote a paper on finding Kaposi's sarcoma in homosexual men who had become infected. Then things began to change of AIDS was reported among the female partners of men who had the disease suggesting it could be passed on via heterosexual sex. Things got worse as the actor Rock Hudson died, and left $250,000 to set up the American Foundation for AIDS Research (amfAR).

In 1982, Willy Rozenbaum, a clinician at the Hôpital Bichat hospital in Paris, asked French virologist, Louis Montagnier for assistance in establishing the cause of this mysterious new syndrome, AIDS. Rozenbaum had suggested at scientific meetings that the cause of the disease might be a retrovirus and knew Montagnier and his colleagues (Françoise Barré-Sinoussi and Jean-Claude Chermann) at the Pasteur Institute, had extensive experience with retroviruses. Montagnier and his team examined samples taken from Rozenbaum's AIDS patients and found the virus that would later become known as HIV in a lymph node biopsy. In May 1983, two papers were published in the same issue of Science, both claiming the same breakthrough: the identification of a virus apparently linked to AIDS. At this time, Montagnier's team called this new virus the 'lymphadenopathy-associated virus', or LAV.

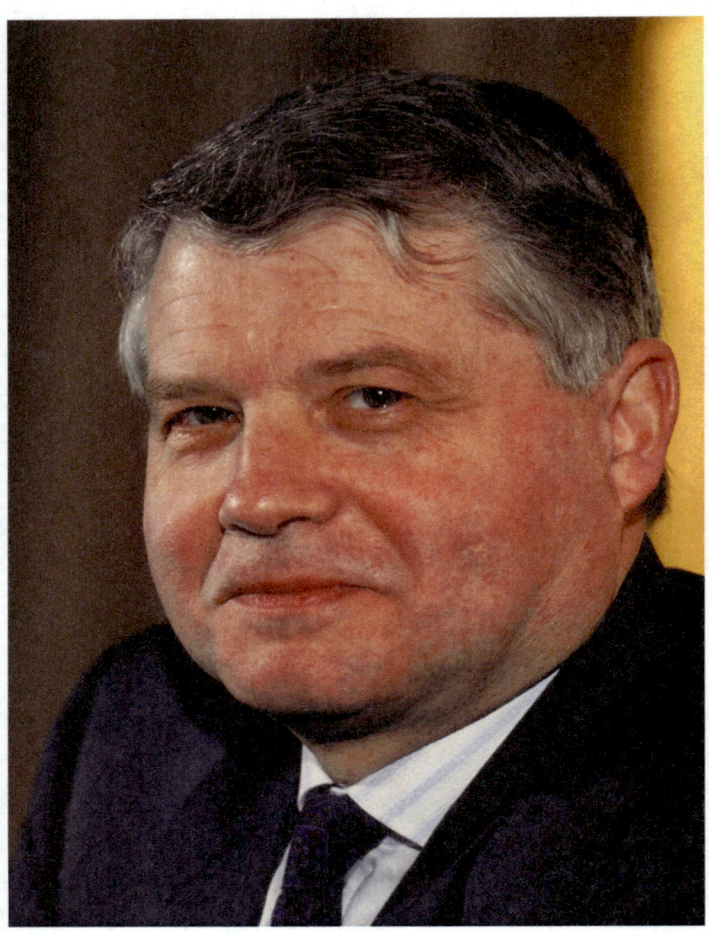

Luc Antoine Montagnier

It was still not known whether this virus was the cause of AIDS. By coincidence, another team led by Robert Gallo of the United States, published another paper in the same issue of Science that provided evidence that this virus caused AIDS. However, Gallo called the virus 'human T-lymphotropic virus type III' (HTLV-III) because of perceived similarities with HTLV-I and II, which had previously been discovered in his lab. This difficulty in two scientists reaching the same conclusion by two different methods led to many years of dispute about whether Montagnier's or Gallo's group was first to isolate who had actually discovered the HIV virus. But the coincidence of two teams making the same claim sparked a bitter row about me between the team leaders, and there was a period where one team accused the other of stealing intellectual property, when I visited California, after being sent there from Paris. As neither team could prove this actually happened, the waiting world waited with bated breath hoping that they would combine forces and seek out a treatment for the pandemic. In the end, further research by the US team confirmed the AIDS connection, and I was ceremoniously named the Human Immunodeficiency Virus (HIV).

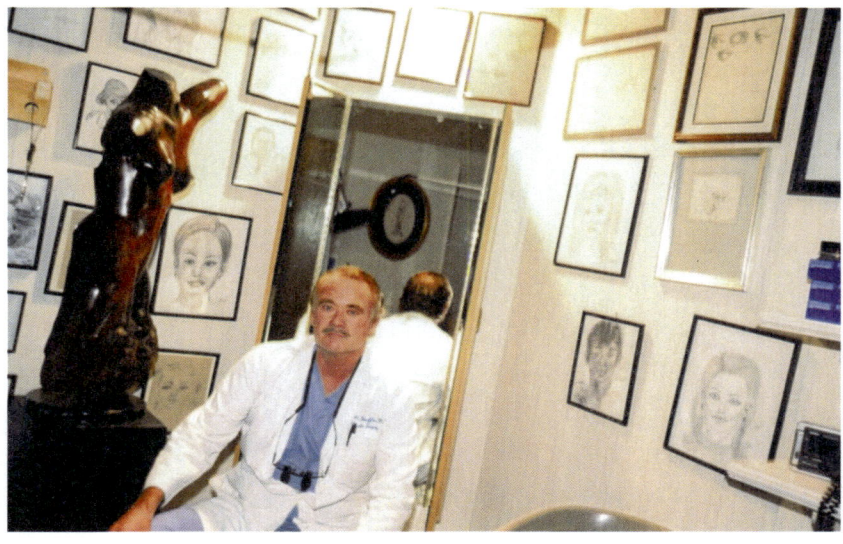

Dr Arnold Klein in Beverly Hills, California on May 19, 2002

In August 1985, Arnold Klein joined the board of the Los Angeles-based National AIDS Research Foundation (NARF). In 2007, Klein founded The Elizabeth Taylor Endowment for the UCLA CARE Centre, a facility that focuses on advancing HIV/AIDS research and treatment. He really was going all out to eliminate me from the planet. The November 2008 issue of L'Uomo Vogue reported that he raised in excess of $274 million for HIV research and care. It certainly was a long way from Kinshasa for me to have come. In 1987, the US and French governments settled that dispute by declaring both teams' co-discoverers. Gallo's team were accused of having wrongfully acquired the virus from the Paris team – a charge later rejected by investigators.

In that year, the FDA also approved the first antiretroviral drug, zidovudine (AZT), as treatment against me. It could also be used to prevent mother-to-child spread during birth or after a needlestick injury or other potential exposure. It was the same year, The Bangles sang 'Walk Like An Egyptian', and Andy Warhol died. But I could easily beat that medicine because even at the highest doses that could be tolerated in patients, it only slowed my replication and progression. It was a bit like slowing down the electricity supply to the rogue worker building iPhones in China, and prolonged AZT treatment led to me developing resistance by mutation of my reverse transcriptase. Two years later the WHO estimated there were up to 400,000 cases worldwide, and people began to panic with the rising number of deaths. One group wanted to hold an AIDS conference in San Francisco, while others, including many members of Congress wanted to ban HIV+ patients from entering America. It took thirty-three years later for the travel ban preventing HIV-positive people from entering the USA to be lifted. By the end of 1990, there were probably a million HIV cases in America, and ten times this number living worldwide.

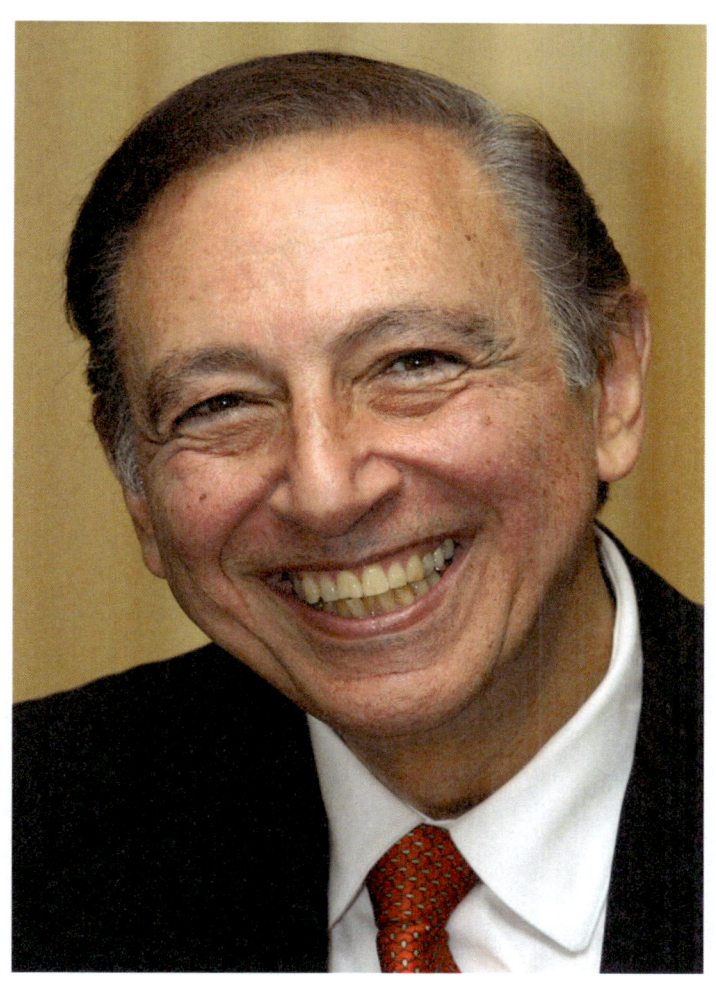

Robert Gallo

The striking similarity between the first two human immunodeficiency virus type 1 (HIV-1) isolates ('lymphadenopathy-associated virus', or LAV, isolated at the Pasteur Institute) and human T-lymphotropic virus type III (HTLV-III), reported to be isolated at the Laboratory of Tumor Cell Biology (LTCB) of the National Cancer Institute) still provoked considerable controversy because other scientists found a high level of variability amongst all subsequent HIV-1 isolates. Eventually, the Office of Scientific Integrity at the National Institutes of Health attempted to clear up the waring scientists by commissioning a group at Roche to look again at old samples from the Pasteur Institute and the Laboratory of

Tumour Cell Biology (LTCB) of the National Cancer Institute that had been analysed between 1983 and 1985. The group was led by Sheng-Yung Chang and Barbara H. Bowman, associated with the University of California who examined old specimens, and concluded in Nature in 1993 that Gallo's virus indeed had come from Montagnier's lab. Chang determined that the French group's LAV was a virus from one patient that had contaminated a culture from another. On request, Montagnier's group had sent a sample of this culture to Gallo, not knowing it contained two viruses.

In June 1995, the FDA approved the first protease inhibitor beginning a new era of highly active antiretroviral treatment (HAART), which meant the use of multiple drugs that act on different viral targets. There is no doubt this hit me hard, the papers showing an immediate decline of between 60% and 80% in rates of AIDS-related deaths and hospitalisation in those countries which could afford it. In 1996, the Joint United Nations Programme on AIDS (UNAIDS) was established to advocate for global action on the epidemic and coordinate the response to HIV and AIDS across the UN. In 1999, the WHO announced that AIDS was the fourth biggest cause of death worldwide and the number one killer in Africa. At this stage, I had infected thirty-three million people and over fourteen million people had died worldwide from AIDS since the time that I arrived in America.

In September 2000, the United Nations adopted the Millennium Development Goals which included a specific goal to reverse the spread of HIV, malaria, and TB. Each goal had specific targets, and dates for achieving those targets. To accelerate progress, the G8 finance ministers agreed to provide enough funds to the World Bank, the (IMF) and the African Development Bank (AfDB) to cancel $40 to $55 billion in debt owed by members of the heavily indebted poor countries to allow them to redirect resources to programs for improving health and education and for alleviating poverty. UNAIDS reported that AIDS was now by far the leading cause of death in sub-Saharan Africa. President George W. Bush announced a $15 billion, five-year plan to combat AIDS, primarily in countries with a high number of HIV infections. In 2011, results from the HPTN 052 trial, and publication in the *New England Journal of Medicine* reduced the risk of HIV transmission by 96% among serodiscordant couples. In 2015, an estimated 35 million people were living with HIV and the number of people in Russia living with HIV reached one million. It is estimated that 65% of all new HIV diagnoses in Europe occurred in Russia. Presently, more than half of the global population living with HIV are receiving antiretroviral treatment.

The UN Millennium Development Goals (MDGs) were eight international development goals for the year 2015 that had been established following the Millennium Summit of the United Nations in 2000, following the adoption of the United Nations Millennium Declaration. All 191 United Nations member states, and at least 22 international organizations, committed to help achieve the following Millennium Development Goals by 2015:

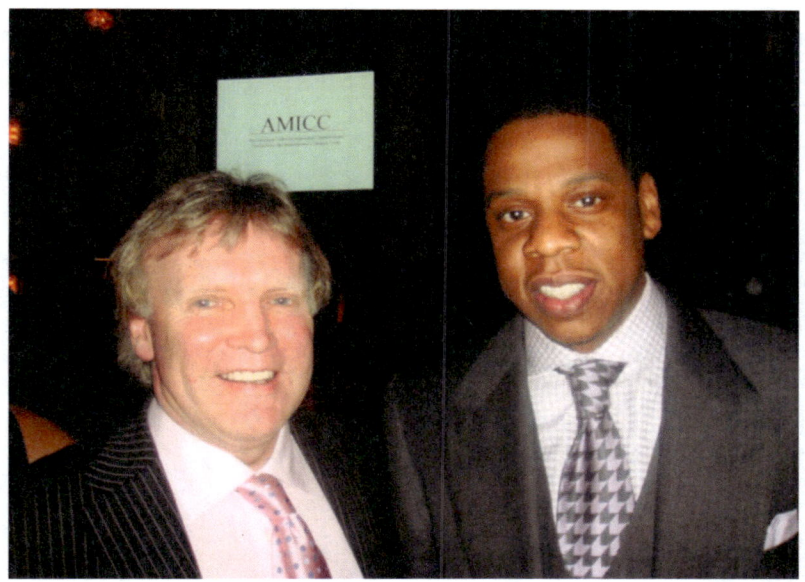

The author with Jay-Z on the United Nations Millennium Development Goals

- To eradicate extreme poverty and hunger
- To achieve universal primary education
- To promote gender equality and empower women
- To reduce child mortality
- To improve maternal health
- To combat HIV/AIDS, malaria, and other diseases
- To ensure environmental sustainability
- To develop a global partnership for development

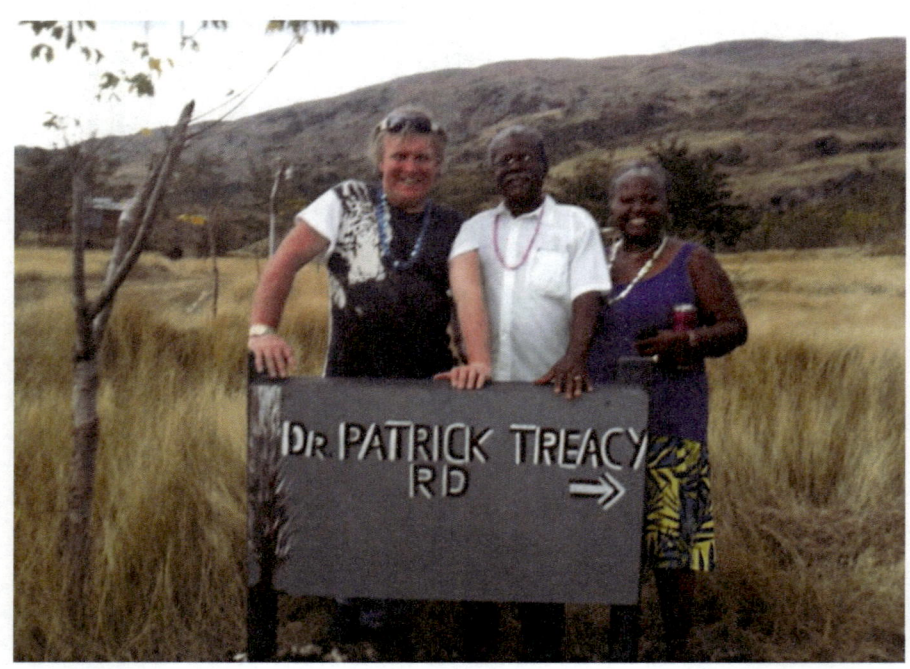

The author with Bishop and Maman Dorcilien in Mirebalais, Haiti. They had previously returned from working in education in the Democratic Republic of the Congo. They were free of any disease.

I Am SARS-Cov-2, the Corona Virus, Who Caused the Worldwide Covid Pandemic

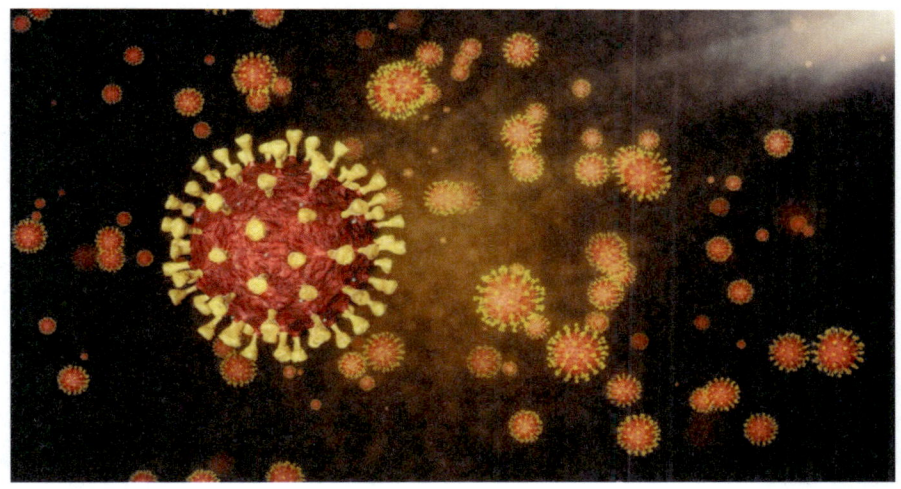

Coronaviruses (CoVs) are positive-stranded RNA viruses with a crown-like appearance under an electron microscope (coronam is the Latin term for crown) due to the presence of spike glycoproteins on the envelope. The most recent common ancestor (MRCA) of all coronaviruses is estimated to have existed as recently as 8000 BCE, although some models place the common ancestor as far back as 55 million years or more, implying long term coevolution with bat and avian species. CoVs are enveloped, positive-stranded RNA viruses with nucleocapsid. In a timeline that reaches the present day, this epidemic of cases with unexplained low respiratory infections was first reported to the WHO Country Office in China, on December 31, 2019. It has since spread like wildfire, leading to nearly 700 million cases, and almost 7 million deaths globally. Its impact on the world has been devastating. Despite significant advancements in clinical research, many countries continue to experience outbreaks of this viral illness, primarily due to the emergence of mutant variants of the virus.

History of SARS-CoV-2.

In December 2019, a cluster of pneumonia cases, of unexplained low respiratory infections was first detected in Wuhan, the largest metropolitan area in China's Hubei province. The Chinese authorities said it was caused by a newly identified β-coronavirus. By 7th January, Chinese scientists rapidly isolated me from a patient and after releasing my genetic sequence, called me SARS-CoV-2. On January 12th, the World Health Organization named me the 2019-novel coronavirus (2019-nCoV) and two weeks later officially declared that my epidemic was a public health emergency of international concern. They said that I was a new highly contagious virus, which had the ability to spread globally. By then, I was in eighteen countries with four countries reporting human-to-human transmission. On February 11, 2020, the WHO Director-General, D Tedros Adhanom Ghebreyesus, announced that the disease I caused was to be called 'COVID-19', which is the acronym of 'coronavirus disease 2019'. Initially, I liked my name 2019-nCoV, but on 11 February 2020, some Coronavirus Study Group (CSG) proposed to name me *SARS-CoV-2*. By now, I was receiving worldwide attention. Subsequently, the task of experts of the International Committee on Taxonomy of Viruses (ICTV) said my new name was going to SARS-CoV-2, as I looked very similar to a cousin that had caused the SARS outbreak of 2003. While related, I was actually quite different. My cousins had indeed wreaked havoc throughout the world before I was born. One had caused a severe acute respiratory syndrome coronavirus (SARS-CoV) that began in Asia in 2002–2003, and a distant cousin H1N1 influenza in 2009, had indeed been recorded. Most recently, my Middle Eastern cousin (MERS-CoV) did something similar in Saudi Arabia in 2012. One WHO member said, "I marked the third introduction of a highly pathogenic and large-scale epidemic coronavirus into the human population in the twenty-first century." Anyway, I soon caused a worldwide sudden and substantial increase in hospitalisations for pneumonia with the multiorgan disease. By March 2020, a total of 79,968 cases of COVID-19 had been confirmed in mainland China including 2873 deaths. Retrospective investigations by Chinese authorities identified while some of the earliest known cases had a link to a wholesale food market in Wuhan, some did not. World governments began work to establish immediate international countermeasures to stem the devastating effects and it has been estimated that by implementing nationwide lockdowns, Europe may have saved at least three million lives across eleven nations.

As the plot thickened, several independent research groups identified that I belonged to a β-coronavirus, with a highly identical genome to bat coronavirus, pointing to bat as my natural home. That meant I used the same receptor key called *angiotensin-converting enzyme 2* (ACE2) as that my cousins to enter the cells along the respiratory tract, and while there to reproduce and send my children out to infect others and basically keep the family alive. Things were marching along steadily, when on February 26, 2020, I crossed the Atlantic and entered the United States (US). Trying to find out where I came from began to be a contentious issue since the earliest reports of my novel disease. Given that many of the earliest cases of pneumonia caused by COVID-19 disease were linked to direct exposure to the Huanan Seafood Wholesale Market of Wuhan, it seemed that spread by direct animal-to-human transmission was the possible cause. However, subsequent cases were not associated with this exposure mechanism and people began to question that I was spread by human-to-human transmission, and this had huge ramifications for human interactions around the globe, especially as it appeared that it could occur from individuals who were totally asymptomatic. The Chinese health authorities shut the Wuhan market down on 1 January 2020, but a clinical study on a cluster of cases reported that of 41 patients whom I had infected bore no direct link to the seafood market. Then an article in *The Lancet* showed that the local Chinese health authority started an epidemiological alert on 31 December 2019; but there was an initial case one month before, which I had infected that had no connection with Wuhan Huanan Seafood Wholesale Market. *The New England Journal of Medicine* indicated that 45% of those whose symptoms started in December 2019 had no connections to the market. The US government under President Donald Trump became openly disparaging about the Chinese authorities' official statement on the origin of the outbreak, and in late April, the US secretary of state Mike Pompeo actually claimed to have seen 'strong evidence' that I originated in a laboratory in Wuhan but never provided any evidence and the world assumed they were not being genuine.

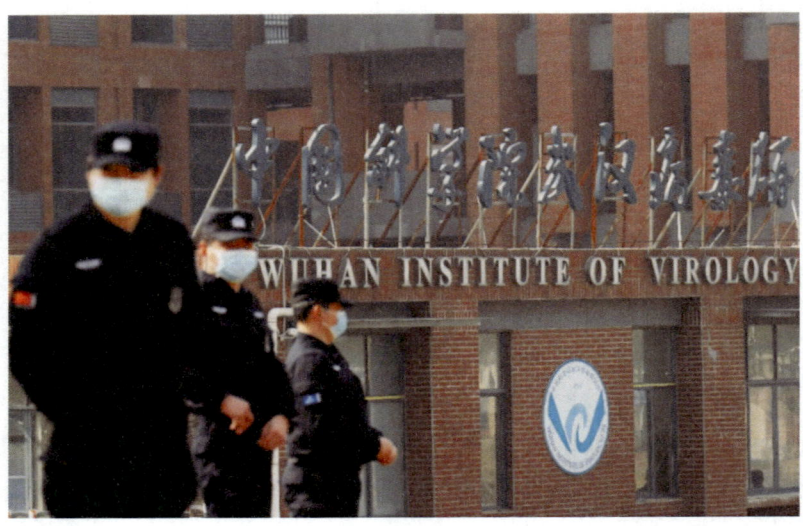

Security personnel keep watch outside Wuhan Institute of Virology during the visit by the World Health Organization (WHO) team tasked with investigating the origins of the coronavirus disease (COVID-19), in Wuhan, Hubei province, China February 3, 2021.

The Wuhan Institute of Virology is a biosafety level 4 (BSL-4) research laboratory located in Jiangxia District, Wuhan, Hubei. It was also built to withstand a magnitude-7 earthquake, even though the region has no history of earthquakes. By coincidence, it has been an active research centre for the study of all my cousins, and has strong ties to the Galveston National Laboratory in the United States, the Centre International de Recherche en Infectiologie in France and the National Microbiology Laboratory in Canada. Many people began to believe the speculation that I escaped from it, either by intent (for use as a bioweapon) or because of a lapse in safety procedures. In this period, Luc Montagnier, a French virologist, who was awarded a Nobel Prize in 2008 for his involvement in the discovery of the HIV family, also endorsed the idea that the virus was man-made as he claimed that I contained sequences from HIV-1. Montagnier was born on August 18, 1932 in Chabris, a village located in Berry south of the Loire Valley.

He was only eight when he witnessed the German invasion of France and had to flee with his parents when they began to bomb his house, beside the railway station. After getting his degree, he moved to Kingsley Sanders' laboratory at Carshalton near London to study the foot and mouth virus.

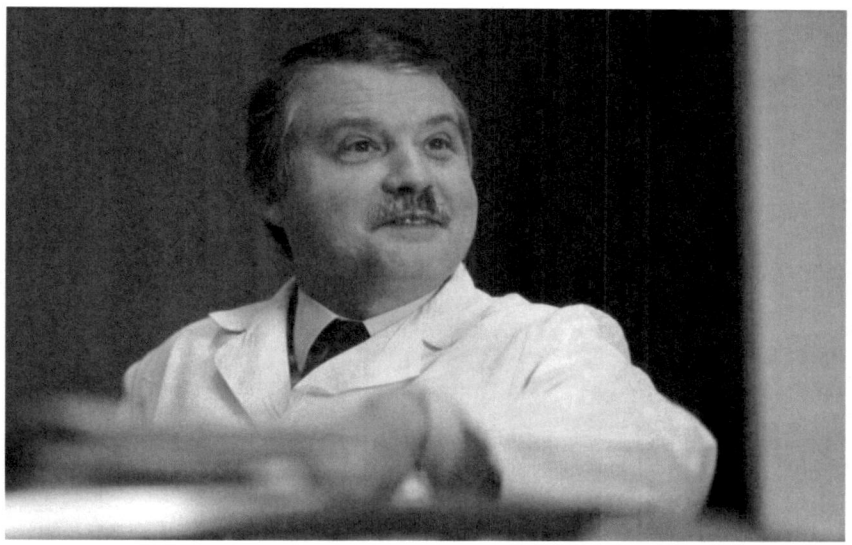

Professor Luc Montagnier portrait at the Pasteur Institute, Institut Pasteur Paris France 1980s

While there, he identified that RNA could replicate like DNA by making a base-paired complementary strand. He eventually went back to work at the Institute Curie in Paris, having spent a period at the new Institute of Virology in Glasgow. In 1969, scientists queried whether a key enzyme was also associated with the oncogenic RNA viruses Montagnier and his team examined samples taken from AIDS patients and found the virus that would later become known as HIV in a lymph node biopsy. In May 1983, two papers appeared in the same issue of Science claimed the same breakthrough: the identification of a virus apparently linked to AIDS. Montagnier's team named it 'lymphadenopathy-associated virus', or LAV, since it was not then clear until Robert Gallo proved it that it was the cause of AIDS. His claim was dismissed as a conspiracy theory, highlighting the lack of evidence that SARS-CoV-2 is an engineered hybrid virus containing HIV-1 sequences. However, mentioning this as a possible aetiology was enough to get me barred from Facebook for a week while writing this article.

Kristian Andersen et al. in a Nature Medicine study, dismiss the idea that I was engineered, proposing my arrival came through natural selection by an

Sanimal host with zoonotic transfer. They conclude that it would be unlikely that the key I use to enter human cells could have been acquired through serial passage in cell lines or animal models, arguing against the idea that my origins was in a laboratory. Zheng-Li Shi et al. at the Wuhan Institute of Virology noted my close similarity to my cousins. Leaving it most probable I mutated while hibernating in a bat.

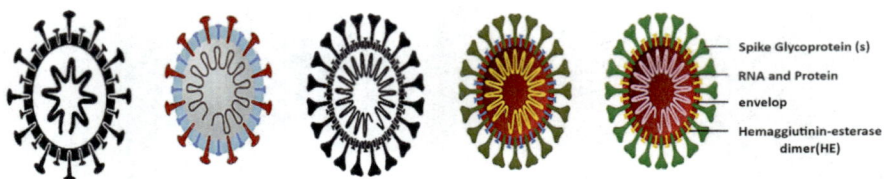

Features, Evaluation, and Treatment of Coronavirus (COVID-19) *

SARS-CoV-2 is prone to genetic evolution resulting in multiple variants that may have different characteristics compared to its ancestral strains. Based on the epidemiological update by the WHO, five SARS-CoV-2 VOCs have been identified since the beginning of the pandemic:

- **Alpha (B.1.1.7):** first variant of concern described in the United Kingdom (UK) in late December 2020
- **Beta (B.1.351)**: first reported in South Africa in December 2020
- **Gamma(P.1)**: first reported in Brazil in early January 2021
- **Delta (B.1.617.2):** first reported in India in December 2020
- **Omicron (B.1.1.529):** first reported in South Africa in November 2021

Clinical Manifestations of COVID-19

The typical incubation period for SARS-CoV-2 is around 5.1 days, with most individuals experiencing symptoms within 11.5 days after being infected.[74] COVID-19 can manifest across a spectrum of clinical presentations, ranging from no symptoms or mild symptoms (paucisymptomatic) to severe illness

---

*Information from Stat Pearls: Features, Evaluation, and Treatment of Coronavirus (COVID-19) Marco Cascella; Michael Rajnik; Arturo Cuomo; Scott C. Dulebohn; Raffaela Di Napoli.

characterized by acute respiratory failure requiring mechanical ventilation, septic shock, and multiple organ failure. It is estimated that approximately 17.9% to 33.3% of infected individuals may remain asymptomatic.

Diagnosis

- Molecular Test: The WHO recommends collecting specimens from both the upper respiratory tract (naso-and oropharyngeal samples) and lower respiratory tract such as expectorated sputum, endotracheal aspirate, or bronchoalveolar lavage. In the laboratory, amplification of the genetic material extracted from the saliva or mucus sample is through.
- A reverse polymerase chain reaction (RT-PCR), which involves the synthesis of a double-stranded DNA molecule from an RNA mold. If the test result is positive, it is recommended that the test is repeated for verification.
- Serology: Despite the numerous antibody tests designed, to date serologic diagnosis has limitations in both specificity and sensitivity.

Laboratory Examinations

- In the early stage of the disease, a normal or decreased total white blood cell count (WBC) and a decreased lymphocyte count can be demonstrated. Interestingly, lymphopenia appears to be a negative prognostic factor.
- Increased values of liver enzymes, lactate dehydrogenase (LDH), muscle enzymes, and C-reactive protein can be detected.
- The elevated neutrophil-to-lymphocyte ratio (NLR), derived NLR ratio (d-NLR) [neutrophil count divided by the result of WBC count minus neutrophil count], and platelet-to-lymphocyte ratio, can be the expression of the inflammatory storm.
- Increased D-dimer.
- In critical patients, D-dimer value is increased, blood lymphocytes decreased persistently, and laboratory alterations of multiorgan imbalance (high amylase, coagulation disorders, etc.) are found.

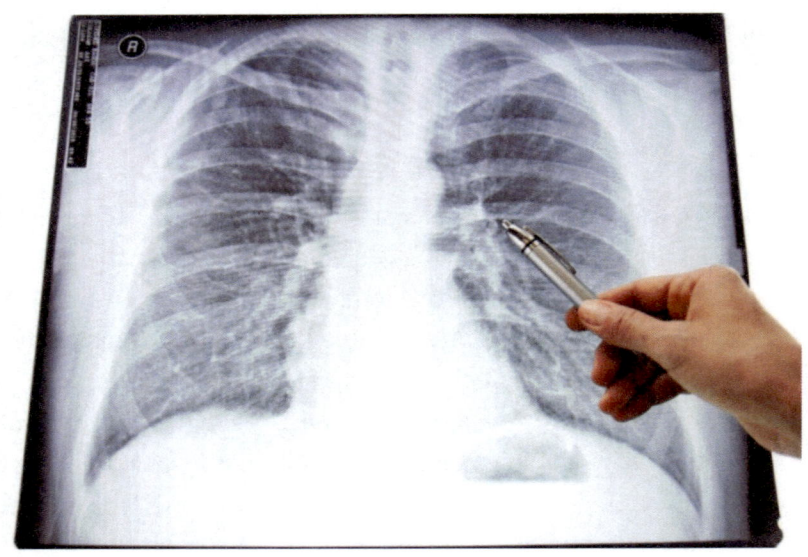

Covid X Ray showing bilateral multifocal alveolar opacities.

Imaging

- Chest X-ray Examination: since the disease manifests itself as pneumonia, radiological imaging has a fundamental role in the diagnostic process, management, and follow-up. Examination generally shows bilateral multifocal alveolar opacities, which tend to confluence up to the complete opacity of the lung. Pleural effusion can be associated.
- Chest Computed Tomography (CT) : given the high sensitivity of the method, in particular high-resolution CT (HRCT), is the method of choice in the study of COVID-19 pneumonia, even in the initial stages. The most common findings are multifocal bilateral 'ground or ground glass' (GG) areas associated with consolidation areas with patchy distribution.
- Lung Ultrasound: Ultrasound can allow evaluating the evolution of the disease, from a focal interstitial pattern up to 'white lung' with evidence often of subpleural consolidations. It should be performed within the first 24 hours in the suspect and every 24/48 hours and can be useful for

patient follow-up, choice of the setting of mechanical ventilation, and for the indication of prone positioning.

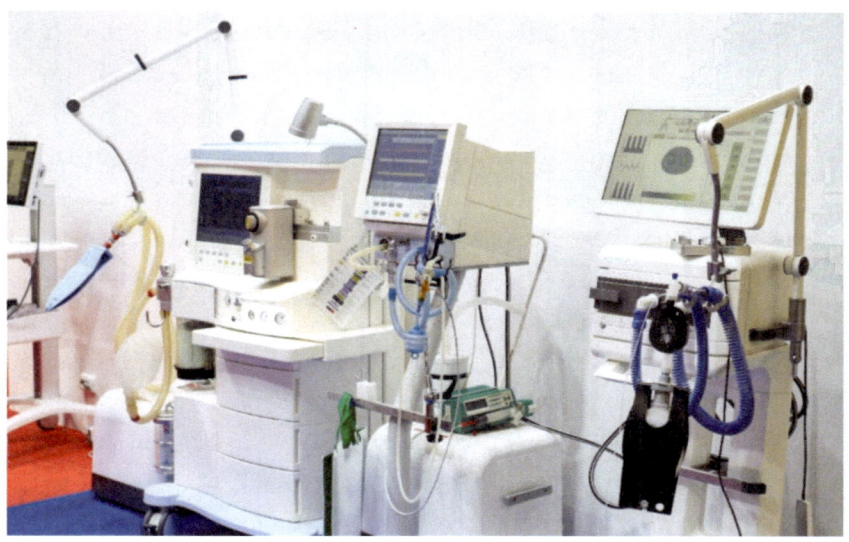

Treatment / Management

There is no specific antiviral treatment recommended for COVID-19, and no vaccine is currently available. The treatment is symptomatic, and oxygen therapy represents the first step for addressing respiratory impairment. Non-invasive (NIV) and invasive mechanical ventilation (IMV) may be necessary in cases of respiratory failure refractory to oxygen therapy. Again, intensive care is needed to deal with complicated forms of the disease.

- **O2 Fast Challenge:** In a patient with a SpO2 < 93–94% (< 88–90% if COPD) or a respiratory rate > 28–30/min, or dyspnoea, the administration of oxygen by a 40% Venturi mask must be performed. After a 5 to 10 minutes reassessment, if the clinical and instrumental picture has improved the patient continues the treatment and undergoes a re-evaluation within 6 hours. In case of failure improvement, or new worsening, the patient undergoes a non-invasive treatment, if not contraindicated.
- **High-Flow Nasal Oxygen (HFNO) and Non-invasive Ventilation:** Because this procedure has a greater risk of aerosolization, it should be used in negative pressure rooms. Indication: when it is difficult to

maintain SpO2 > 92% and/or not improved dyspnoea through standard oxygen. Switch to NIV if the symptomatology is not improved after 1 hour with flow > 50 L/min and FiO2 > 70%.
- **Non-invasive ventilation and Continuous Positive Airway Pressure:** NIV/CPAP has a key role in managing COVID-19-associated respiratory failure.
- **Intubation and Protective Mechanical Ventilation:** Special precautions are necessary during intubation. The procedure should be executed by an expert operator who uses personal protective equipment (PPE) such as an FFP3 or N95 mask, protective goggles, disposable gown long sleeve raincoat, disposable double socks, and gloves. If possible, rapid sequence intubation (RSI) should be performed. Preoxygenation (100% O2 for 5 minutes) should be performed via the continuous positive airway pressure (CPAP) method. Heat and moisture exchanger (HME) must be positioned between the mask and the circuit of the fan or between the mask and the ventilation balloon.

ARDS (Acute Respiratory Distress Syndrome) is a condition marked by the sudden onset of severe respiratory failure or the worsening of an existing respiratory condition. Its diagnosis requires the evaluation of specific clinical and ventilatory criteria, including the use of chest imaging techniques such as chest radiography, CT scan, or lung ultrasound. These imaging methods aim to identify bilateral opacities (lung infiltrates > 50%) that cannot be fully explained by effusions, lobar abnormalities, or lung collapse.

Mild ARDS: 200 mmHg < PaO2/FiO2 ≤ 300 mmHg in patients not receiving mechanical ventilation or in those managed through non-invasive ventilation (NIV) by using positive end-expiratory pressure (PEEP) or a continuous positive airway pressure (CPAP) ≥ 5 cmH2O.

Moderate ARDS: 100 mmHg < PaO2/FiO2 ≤ 200 mmHg

Severe ARDS: PaO2/FiO2 ≤ 100 mmHg.

Other Therapies

- **Corticosteroids:** Among other therapeutic strategies, although systemic corticosteroids for the treatment of viral pneumonia or acute respiratory distress syndrome (ARDS) were not recommended, in severe CARDS these drugs are usually used (e.g., methylprednisolone 1 mg/Kg/day).
- **Antiviral Agents: Some** antiviral treatments have been approved, including These include: Paxlovid—an oral medicine taken as tablets and Sotrovimab—given through a drip in your arm (infusion). Other approaches include lopinavir/ritonavir (400/100 mg orally every 12 hours). Preclinical studies suggested that remdesivir (GS5734)—an inhibitor of RNA polymerase with in vitro activity against multiple RNA viruses, including Ebola—could be effective for both prophylaxis and therapy of HCoVs infections.
- Several anti-flu drugs such as oseltamivir have been used for the treatment of COVID-19 patients. Another anti-flu medication, favipiravir demonstrated a certain efficacy against SARS-CoV-2 in vitro.
- **Antiviral/Immunomodulatory Drugs:** Chloroquine (500 mg every 12 hours), and hydroxychloroquine (200 mg every 12 hours) were proposed during the Covid pandemic as potential immunomodulatory therapy. Gautret showed that hydroxychloroquine reduced viral load and this effect was enhanced by the macrolides azithromycin but WHO and most hospitals do not recommend this treatment.
- **Serotherapy:** Antibodies taken from the blood of healed individuals represent a therapeutic option currently under study. It is calculated that the dose of antibodies necessary for the treatment of a single patient with SARS-CoV-2, requires the removal of antibodies carried out by at least three patients recovered from the SARS-CoV-2 infection. A clinical trial was launched (June 11, 2020) for investigating an antibody cocktail for the prevention and treatment of COVID-19.
- **Anticoagulant:** Because COVID-19 patients have a higher incidence of venous thromboembolism and anticoagulant therapy is associated with reduced ICU mortality, it is suggested that patients should receive thromboprophylaxis. Moreover, in the case of known thrombophilia or

thrombosis, full therapeutic-intensity anticoagulation (e.g., enoxaparin 1 mg/kg twice daily) is indicated.

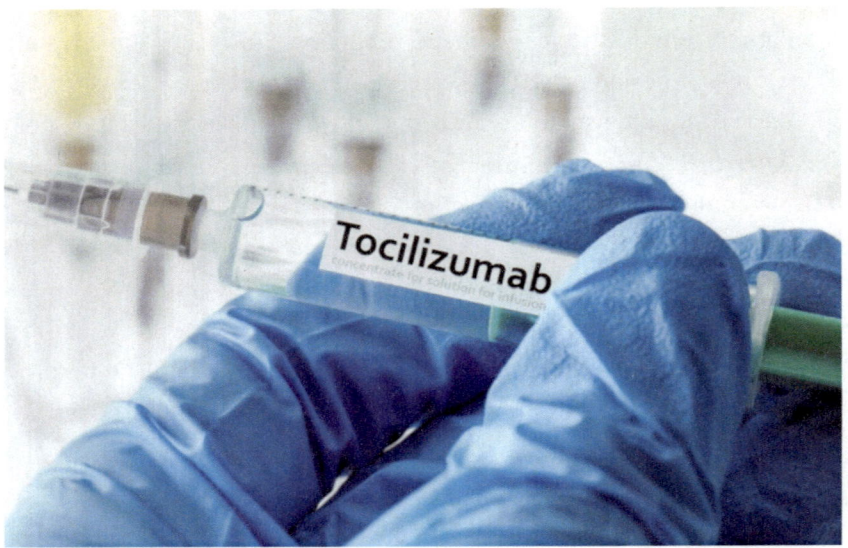

- **Inflammation Inhibitors:** Tocilizumab is a humanized IgG1 monoclonal antibody, directed against the IL-6 receptor and commonly used in the treatment of rheumatoid arthritis, juvenile arthritis, giant cell arthritis, Castleman's syndrome, and for managing toxicity due to immune checkpoint inhibitors. Acalabrutinib is a selective Bruton tyrosine kinase inhibitor, which regulates macrophage signalling and activation.

Other Therapies

When the disease results in complex clinical pictures of MOD, organ function support in addition to respiratory support, is mandatory. Extracorporeal membrane oxygenation (ECMO) for patients with refractory hypoxemia despite lung-protective ventilation should merit consideration after a case-by-case analysis. It can be suggested for those with poor results to prone position ventilation.

Extrapulmonary Manifestations

Although SARS-CoV-2, the virus responsible for COVID-19, primarily affects the respiratory system, it can be considered a systemic viral illness due to the involvement of multiple organs.

- Renal manifestations include the risk of kidney injury, often presenting as acute kidney injury (AKI).

- Cardiac manifestations encompass myocardial injury such as myocardial ischemia/infarction (MI) and myocarditis, along with other common conditions like acute coronary syndrome (ACS), arrhythmias, cardiomyopathy, and cardiogenic shock.

- Haematologic manifestations involve laboratory abnormalities like lymphopenia, thrombocytopenia, leukopenia, elevated ESR levels, C-reactive protein (CRP), lactate dehydrogenase (LDH), and leucocytosis.

- Gastrointestinal manifestations consist of symptoms such as diarrhoea, nausea/vomiting, anorexia, and abdominal pain.

- Hepatobiliary manifestations involve elevated liver function tests, specifically an acute increase in AST and ALT. Endocrinologic manifestations are more severe in patients with underlying disorders like diabetes mellitus.

- Neurologic manifestations include symptoms like headache, stroke, impaired consciousness, seizure disorder, and toxic metabolic encephalopathy.

- Cutaneous manifestations encompass acral lesions resembling pseudo chilblains, erythematous maculopapular rash, vesicular rashes, and urticarial rashes, as observed in patients with COVID-19.

Ugur Sahin. Discover of the Pfizer Covid vaccine

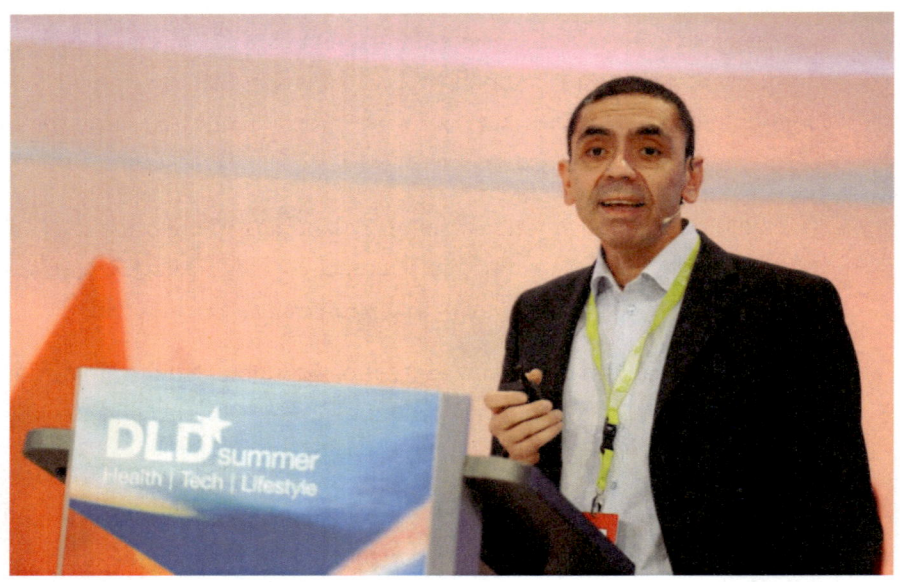

Ugur Sahin (BioNTech AG) DLDsummer15 Conference in Munich, (2015)

Ugur Şahin was born in Iskenderun, Turkey. When he was four years old, his family immigrated to Germany, where his father worked in a Ford car factory. In 1990, he graduated from University of Cologne, with a degree in medicine. In 1993, obtained a PhD in immunology from the same university. In 2000, Sahin joined the faculty of the University of Mainz, and the next year founded Ganymed Pharmaceuticals, which developed cancer cancer-fighting antibodies. In 2006, Sahin became a professor of oncology at the University of Mainz. Drs Sahin and his wife Tuereci co-founded BioNTech, a German biotechnology company dedicated to the development and manufacture of active immunotherapies for the treatment of serious diseases. Their research work was based on messenger RNA (mRNA) for use as individualized cancer immunotherapies, as vaccines against infectious diseases and as protein replacement therapies for rare diseases. The Bill & Melinda Gates Foundation has invested $55 (£41.8) million in the company, which also works on HIV and tuberculosis programmes.

In 2018, Dr Sahin gave a lecture at an infectious disease conference in Berlin and said his company might be able to use its so-called messenger RNA technology to rapidly develop a vaccine in the event of a global pandemic. Covid-19 did not yet exist, and it had never brought a product to market. Then came the present coronavirus pandemic. In 2020, Pfizer, who had previously collaborated with BioNTech on flu vaccines said they would pay $185m upfront toward the development of the proposed Covid-19 vaccine. The BioNTech vaccine pioneered an entirely new technology that involved injecting part of the virus's genetic code to train the immune system. The vaccine trials, enrolled 30,000 healthy adults, were conducted in several cities in the U.S, and results showed 90% efficacy. In 2020, it became one of the world's lead vaccines for preventing COVID-19 infections, BNT2b2, passed Phase III clinical trials in the United States. Pfizer and BioNTech and provided 200 million doses of their Covid-19 vaccine candidate to the European Union. the largest order for the potential vaccine to date. Ugur Sahin was awarded the Mustafa Prize, a science and technology award, granted by Iran to top researchers and scientists from the Organisation of Islamic Cooperation (OIC) member states. Oezlem Tuereci, is the wife of Dr Ugur Sahin and co-founder and chief medical officer of BioNTech, president of the Association for Cancer Immunotherapy (CIMT), chair of the Cluster for Individualized Immune Intervention (Ci3) and lecturer at the University of Mainz. Türeci is considered a pioneer in cancer immunotherapy. He and his wife now figure among the 100 richest Germans, according to German newspaper Welt am Sonntag. Türeci has been married to Ugur Şahin since 2002, and they have a teenage daughter together.

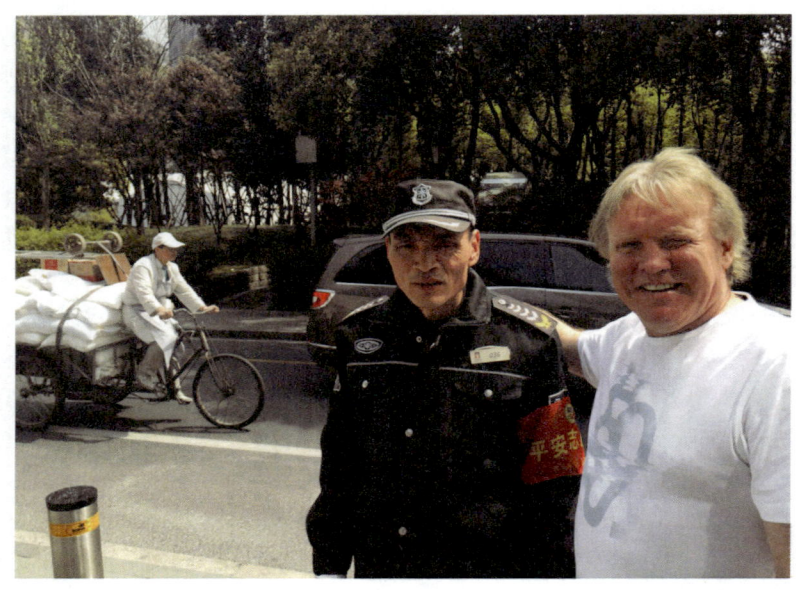

The author in Wuhan before the Covid outbreak

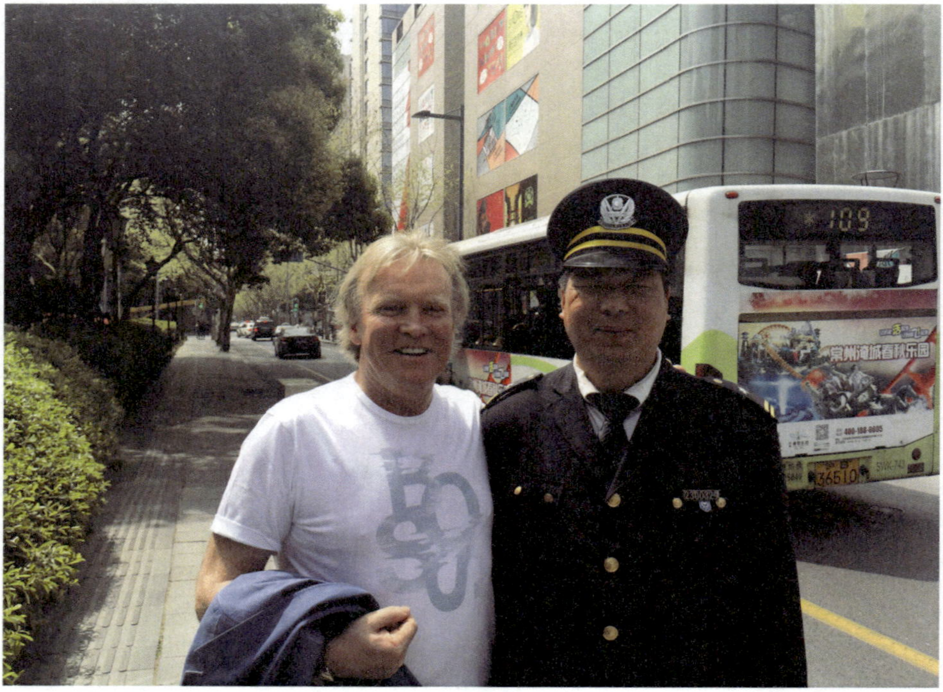

Bacteria

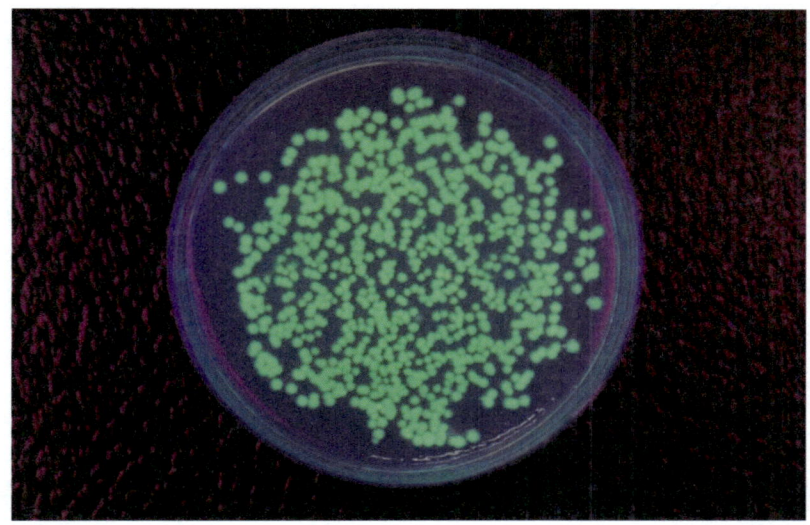

What are bacteria?

Bacteria are single celled microbes. The cell structure is simpler than that of other organisms as there have no nucleus or membrane bound organelles and their data control centre is contained in a single loop of nucleic acid (DNA), containing the genetic information. Some bacteria have an extra circle of genetic material called a plasmid. The plasmid is a small, extrachromosomal DNA molecule within a cell that is separate from chromosomal DNA and can replicate independently, often containing genes that give the microbe some advantage over other bacteria. For example, it may contain a gene that makes the bacterium resistant to a certain antibiotic. Bacteria come in many shapes and sizes, from minute spheres, cylinders, and spiral threads, to flagellated rods, and filamentous chains and are classified accordingly. This gives us spherical (*cocci*), rod (*bacilli*), spiral (*spirilla*), comma (*vibrios*) or corkscrew (spirochaetes). They can exist as single cells, in pairs, chains or clusters. Bacteria are found in every habitat on earth: soil, rock, oceans and even in the polar ice caps. They live in or on other organisms including plants and animals including humans. There are approximately ten times as many bacterial cells as human cells in the human body, many which work for our benefit.

How were bacteria discovered?

Bacteria were first observed by Antoine van Leeuwenhoek in 1676, using a single-lens microscope of his own design. He called them 'animalcules' and published his observations in a series of letters to the Royal Society. Our bodies are home to an estimated 100 trillion 'good' bacteria, many of which reside in the 'microbiome' of our gut. There are also many bacteria present in the microbiome of our skin. Not only do we live in harmony with these beneficial bacteria, but they are actually essential to our survival. In answering the question, are bacteria animals or plants, we can deduce that bacteria are unique organisms and deserve their own separate classification system. Bacteria are neither animals nor plants.

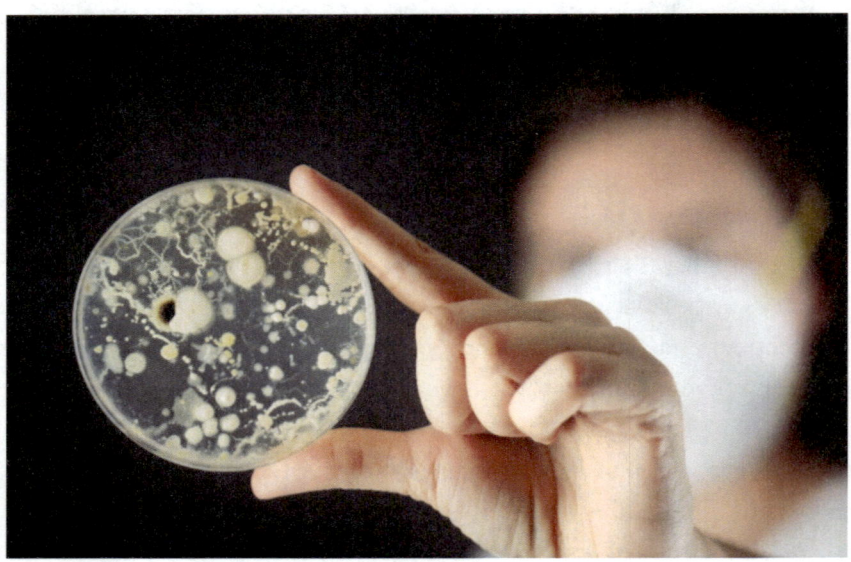

Benefits of Bacteria

Creating products, such as ethanol and enzymes.
Making drugs, such as antibiotics and vaccines.
Making biogas, such as methane.
Cleaning up oil spills and toxic wastes.
Killing plant pests.

Transferring normal genes to human cells in gene therapy.
Fermenting foods.

How do bacteria reproduce?

Bacteria reproduce by binary fission. In this process, the single cell bacterium, divides into two identical daughter cells. The bacterial cell elongates and splits into two daughter cells each with identical DNA to the parent cell. Each daughter cell is a clone of the parent cell. When conditions are favourable, such as the right temperature and nutrients are available, some bacteria like Escherichia coli can divide every 20 minutes. This means that in just seven hours one bacterium can generate 2,097,152 bacteria. After one more hour, the number of bacteria will have risen to a colossal 16,777,216. That's why we can quickly become ill when pathogenic microbes invade our bodies.

How do bacteria cause disease?

Bacteria cause disease by secreting or excreting toxins (as in botulism), by producing toxins internally, which are released when the bacteria disintegrate (as in typhoid), or by inducing sensitivity to their antigenic properties (as in tuberculosis). Viral infections need a host to survive, and they multiply by attaching to cells. Viruses are more dangerous than bacteria as they do cause diseases. In some infections, like pneumonia and diarrhoea, it's difficult to determine whether it was caused by bacteria or a virus and testing may be required. Bacterial infections are most often treated with antibiotics, medications that affect bacterial growth, by either stopping bacteria from multiplying or killing them outright. They do this by attacking the bacteria cell wall or coating (penicillin), or also interfering with bacteria reproduction. Even without antibiotics, most people can fight off a bacterial infection, especially if symptoms are mild. About 70 percent of the time, symptoms of acute bacterial sinus infections go away within two weeks without antibiotics. Bacterial infections may be the result of 'secondary infection' (meaning that the virus initiated the process but a bacteria followed) when the symptoms persist longer than the expected 10–14 days a virus tends to last.

I Am Bacillus Anthracis, 'Deliverer of the Jews to the Promised Land'

Bacillus anthracis is a gram-positive, rod-shaped bacteria that causes the infectious disease known as anthrax. Anthrax occurs naturally in soil and is commonly associated with livestock, such as cattle, sheep, and goats. The bacteria can form spores that are highly resistant and can survive in the environment for long periods. Anthrax can infect humans through contact with infected animals or their products, such as wool, hides, or meat. It can also be transmitted through inhalation of spores or through skin contact with contaminated materials. The severity of the disease depends on the route of exposure.

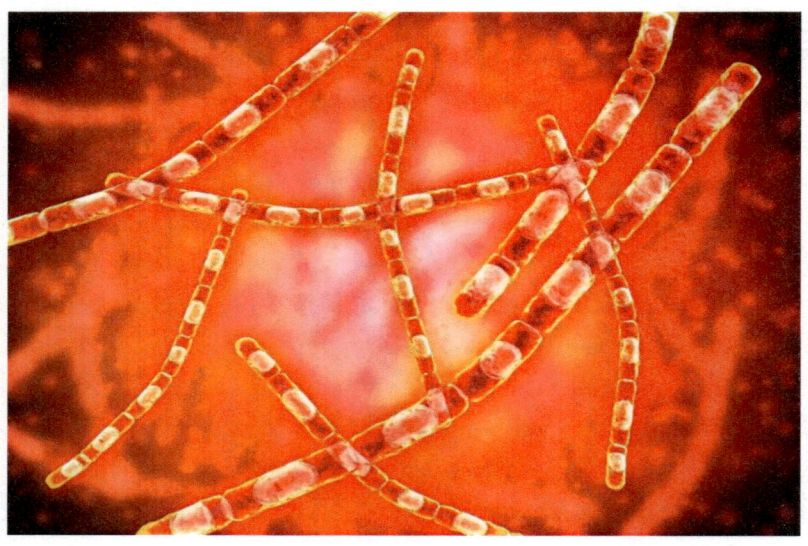

Bacillus anthracis

There are three main forms of anthrax infection: cutaneous anthrax, inhalation anthrax, and gastrointestinal anthrax. Cutaneous anthrax is the most common form and occurs when the bacteria enter through a cut or abrasion on the skin. It typically presents as a painless ulcer with a black centre. Inhalation anthrax is the most severe form and results from inhaling spores into the lungs. It can cause severe respiratory distress and is often fatal if not treated early. Gastrointestinal anthrax occurs from consuming contaminated meat and affects the digestive system. Anthrax is diagnosed through laboratory tests, including culture and identification of the bacteria from samples taken from the affected site or blood. Treatment involves antibiotics, such as ciprofloxacin, doxycycline, or penicillin, along with supportive care. Anthrax has not been characterized as a pandemic in recent history. Anthrax outbreaks have occurred in various parts of the world, with notable historical cases causing significant morbidity and mortality. One example of a significant anthrax epidemic occurred in 1770 in what is now Haiti, resulting in the deaths of approximately 15,000 people. However, it's important to note that this epidemic happened in a specific region rather than being a global pandemic. However, I've decided to include Anthrax has been in the news due to various reasons. One significant event that brought anthrax into the spotlight was the Amerithrax or Anthrax Investigation, which occurred soon after the terrorist attacks of September 11, 2001. This investigation involved a series of biological attacks using anthrax spores, making it one of the largest bioterrorism incidents in U.S. history. Anthrax is considered a potential agent for bioterrorism due to its high infectivity and the ability to cause severe illness even with a small amount of the bacteria. This threat of an anthrax attack has raised concerns regarding public health and national security.

This is my story.

I am Bacillus anthracis, a literary type of bacterium that gets its name from anthracis, (Greek: coal), a reference to the legendary coal-black scabs that I leave behind on some of my victims. I say literary type because my exploits have been reported as the fifth plague of Egypt in the Bible, the sixth plague in the Book of Exodus, the plague in Homer's Iliad, and I am even lamented by Virgil in his novels of ancient Rome. I could have had a hat trick if Shakespeare would have a lived another couple of years later and witnessed the 'Black Bane', that awful plague that killed 60,000 people and many more domestic and wild animals in Europe during the 1600s. Well, now you know, that was me as well!

I was telling you about my exploits during the fifth plague of Egypt (Exodus 9:3)! You know, to be fair, I really feel guilty about that one, because many tried to make me responsible for the present Middle East conflict and even indirectly for Al Qaeda's eventual destruction of the Twin Towers in New York. It is true that in 1998, Al Qaeda leader Osama bin Laden had openly declared that acquiring and using me as a weapon of mass destruction (WMD) was his Islamic duty—an integral part of his jihad. It is also true that immediately after the 2001 anthrax attacks, White House officials did pressurise FBI Director Robert Mueller to publicly blame them on al-Qaeda but it would really be a bit ironic, that present-day Salafiya Islamic fundamentalists from the land of the Pharaohs would now try and use me in their present endeavour of revivalism and hope to bring down Judaeo-Christian America because I actually started that trouble thousands of years before.

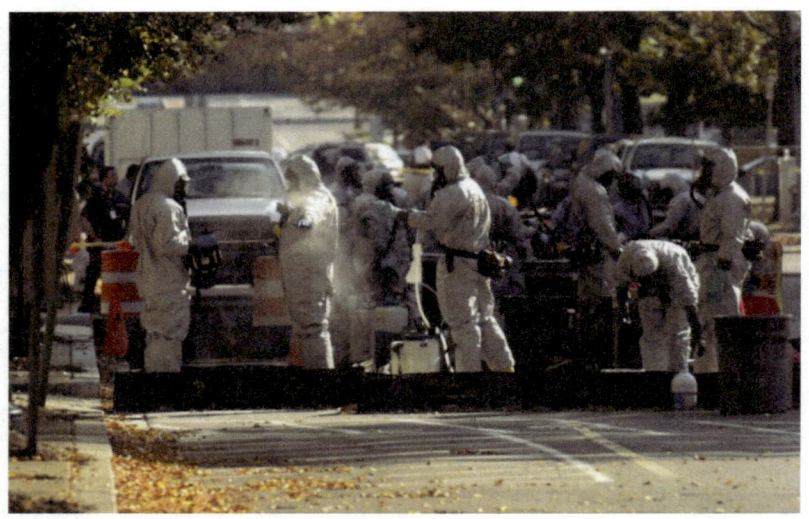

2001 anthrax attacks in America

Because in the good book it says that God told Moses to confront the Pharaoh and tell him to let the Hebrews go, or terrible pestilence would visit the Pharaoh's fields "upon the horses, upon the donkeys, upon the camels, upon the herds and flocks: There shall be a very grievous moraine. And the Lord did that thing on the morrow and all the cattle of Egypt died: but the cattle of the children of Israel died not one." Yes, it was also me who finally convinced the obstinate Pharaoh to release the ancient Hebrews, after a series of other devastating plagues, back in 1300 B.C. The first ones turned the river Nile to blood red and made it undrinkable. The later ones caused the destruction of all the first-born of Egypt in a single night. Then came swarms of frogs invaded the land of Egypt, infesting homes, and surroundings. No sooner had that ended than dust from the ground transformed into lice, covering humans and animals alike. Then swarms of flies or gnats plagued the people and animals, making life difficult. However, it took me, the fifth plague, which killed all the cattle in Egypt, to convince him to let the Hebrews go. Well, to be fair, being the bacterium of both the Virgil and the Iliad, I couldn't be bothered making friends with any those Jewish livestock as they grazed in the poorer ground. The upshot of it all was that the Pharaoh became convinced that their God had spared their cattle and let them go wandering back to the land of Canaan. Well, they made their way back to the land of Canaan, much to the distress of the Pharaoh's descendants.

So, let's speed up through the centuries to the dear old Clausthalian physician, Robert Koch. Robert was born the same year that Richard Wagner wrote 'The Flying Dutchman' and astounded his parents at the age of five by telling them that he could read the newspaper. He completed his MD in 1866 and went to Berlin to study under Virchow. Now, to leave the subject for a while let me tell you about Dr Virchow, who may have singlehandedly caused World War 1, the assassination at Sarajevo of Archduke Franz Ferdinand of Austria, which is always blamed. I will get back to Dr Virchow later. In 1862, Koch went to the University of Göttingen to study medicine, and while there his professor of anatomy was Henle, who published a paper, stating that infectious diseases were caused by living, parasitic organisms. They were getting better at science and before long, I knew they would discover me. It was the same year that another scientific genius, the Frenchman, Louis Pasteur graduated from high school. It was a momentous time of change in Germany, as Prince William became King of Prussia in 1861. It was the same year that Abraham Lincoln became the 16th U.S. President. In 1871, Bismarck united Prussia with surrounding German states to create a new German Empire and Koch volunteered to become the District Medical Officer for Wollstein to do his bit for the Fatherland in the Franco-Prussian War. Being bored in his little flat in the long French evenings, he took to working out why anthrax was so prevalent among the livestock of the village. Koch set to work, inoculating mice (by slivers of wood), with anthrax bacilli taken from the spleens of farm animals that had died of anthrax.

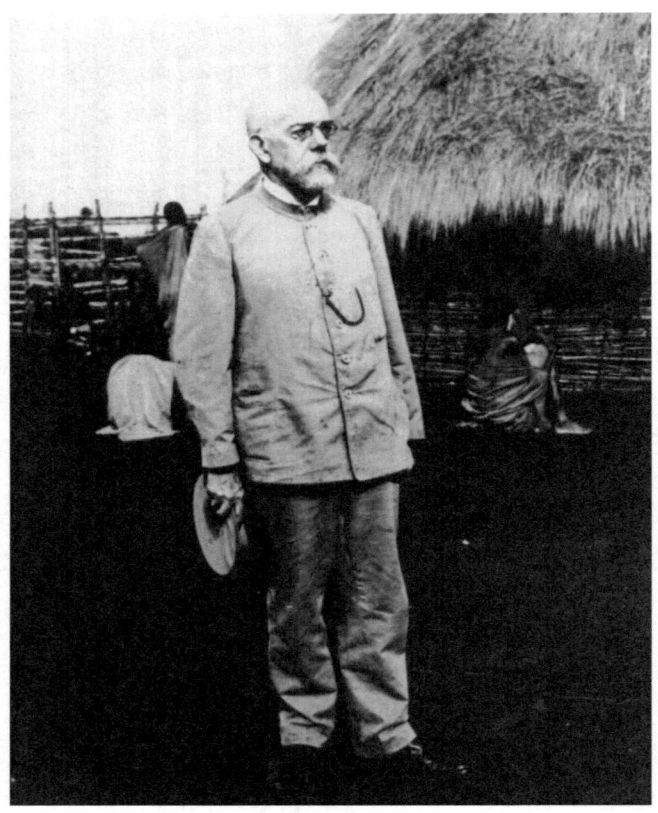

ROBERT KOCH German physician 1843–1910 who isolated Anthrax

He found that the bacilli killed all the mice, but mice that were inoculated with blood from the spleens of healthy animals did not suffer from the disease. This confirmed that the blood of animals suffering from anthrax transmitted the disease. He then grew pure cultures of the bacilli (by growing them on the aqueous humour of an ox's eye) and showed that the organisms could cause anthrax, even if they had had no contact with any kind of animal. He had little equipment in a small flat except for a microscope, which was given to him by his wife, and from that, he laid down the conditions, known as Koch's postulates, which must be satisfied before it can be accepted a particular bacterium causes a particular disease. It was in Wollstein that Koch carried out the research on anthrax, which was at that time prevalent among the farm animals in the district.

Pollender, Rayer and Davaine had already discovered the anthrax bacillus but never proved scientifically that this was the cause of the disease.

Pasteur was studying anthrax at the same time and was developing an attenuated culture to protect animals against infection. Koch under the advice of Professor Cohn, at Breslau, published his findings in 1876. Koch went back to Wollstein and continued his work, inventing new methods of cultivating bacteria on solid media such as potato or agar. He also developed new methods of staining bacteria, which made them more easily visible and helped to identify them and laid down Koch's postulates. He moved to Berlin and in 1882, he published his classical work on the tubercle bacillus. One year later, he went to Egypt to investigate an outbreak of cholera and discovered the vibrio that causes the disease. He also discovered that *haemophilus aegyptius* was the cause of Egyptian ophthalmia. In 1884, he studied more cholera in India and formulated rules for the control of epidemics, which are still used today. His work on cholera, (for which a prize of 100,000 German marks was awarded to him) had an important influence on plans for the conservation of water supplies.

Louis Pasteur was born in Dole, Jura, France, the only son of a tanner who was a sergeant in Napoleon's army. He graduated from college at Besancon in 1840 and two years later gained a BSc. At the age of 26, he became an assistant to Antoine Balard. His research project involved crystallising several different compounds found in the sediments of fermenting wine. He first looked at the crystals of tartaric and paratartaric acid, refusing to accept that the two compounds had the same chemical composition as they rotated polarised light in different directions. He quickly showed one type was the mirror image of the other and by mixing the solutions the substance became inactive. This simple experiment proved that organic molecules with the same chemical composition can exist in space in unique stereospecific forms. Pasteur proposed that asymmetrical molecules were only found in living organisms. We know today that all the proteins of higher animals are made up of only those amino acids that exist in the left-hand form. The mirror image right-hand amino acids are not used by human or animal cells. Likewise, our cells burn only the right-hand form of sugar, not the left-hand form that can be made in the test tube. It was the discovery of asymmetry of organic molecules that provided Pasteur with the evidence to solve his next problem, that of alcoholic fermentation.

In 1854, he was appointed professor of chemistry at the Faculty of Sciences in Lille, an industrial town with several distilleries and factories. In the summer of 1856, M. Bigot, father of one of his students in chemistry, called upon him to help him overcome difficulties he was having manufacturing alcohol by fermentation of beetroot. His fermentations were yielding lactic acid instead of alcohol. Scientists of the period considered fermentation to be simply the chemical breakdown of sugar into the desired molecules. Yeast cells found in the fermenting vats of wine were mostly regarded as by-products or catalytic agents. Pasteur found three clues that allowed him to solve the puzzle.

First, when alcohol was produced normally, the yeast cells were plump and budding. But when lactic acid would form instead of alcohol, small rod-like microbes were always mixed with the yeast cells. Second, analysis of the batches of alcohol showed that amyl alcohol and other complex organic compounds were being formed during the fermentation.

Third, some of these compounds rotated light, that is they were asymmetric. Pasteur suspected that only living cells produced asymmetrical compounds and concluded that yeast was responsible for forming alcohol from sugar and that contaminating microorganisms turned the fermentations sour. He showed that if he heated wine, beer, milk to moderately high temperatures for a few minutes, he could kill the microorganisms and thereby sterilise the batches. If pure cultures of microbes and yeasts were added to sterile mashes uniform, predictable fermentations would follow. Pasteur then conducted a series of ingenious experiments that destroyed the argument supporting 'spontaneous generation'. The experimental design that clinched the argument was the use of the swan-neck flask. In this experiment, fermentable juice was placed in a flask and after sterilisation, the neck was heated and drawn out as a thin tube and sealed. If the flask was opened, air entered but the dust was trapped on the wet walls of the neck and the contents remained sterile, showing that air alone could not trigger the growth of microorganisms. If the flask was tipped to allow the sterile liquid to touch the contaminated walls and this liquid was then returned to the broth, the growth of microorganisms immediately began.

It was a hot summer and Pasteur returned to Paris, leaving the cholera cultures on the shelves of the Arbois Laboratory. When he returned, he discovered that the cultures no longer killed injected chickens. The group set to work to make new cultures of the bacillus and tested these batches on new birds and those healthy previously treated birds. The results were astonishing: The previously injected birds were unaffected by the bacillus, while the new birds all died. When Pasteur saw these results, he immediately realised that in a sense he was repeating the studies of Jenner 80 years earlier who had conferred on humans' immunity to smallpox by vaccinating individuals with a mild form of cowpox. He manufactured chicken cholera vaccines and prevented the disease. He then considered the possibility that attenuated anthrax bacillus might render sheep immune to anthrax. He used various techniques by subjecting the anthrax bacillus to oxidation and even aging and eventually produced a working vaccine.

His results were treated with scepticism and he was challenged by the well-known veterinarian, Rossignol, to conduct a carefully controlled public test of his anthrax vaccine. This was to take place at Pouilly le Fort, a farm in the town of Melun south of Paris. Twenty-five sheep were to be controlled, the other twenty-five were to be vaccinated by Pasteur and then all animals would receive a lethal dose of anthrax. All of the control sheep must die, and the vaccinated sheep must live. When Pasteur's colleagues learned that he had agreed to the test, they were concerned. The challenge was severe and there was no room for error. The vaccines were still in the developmental stage. "What succeeded with 14 sheep in our laboratory will succeed with 50 at Melun," said Pasteur.

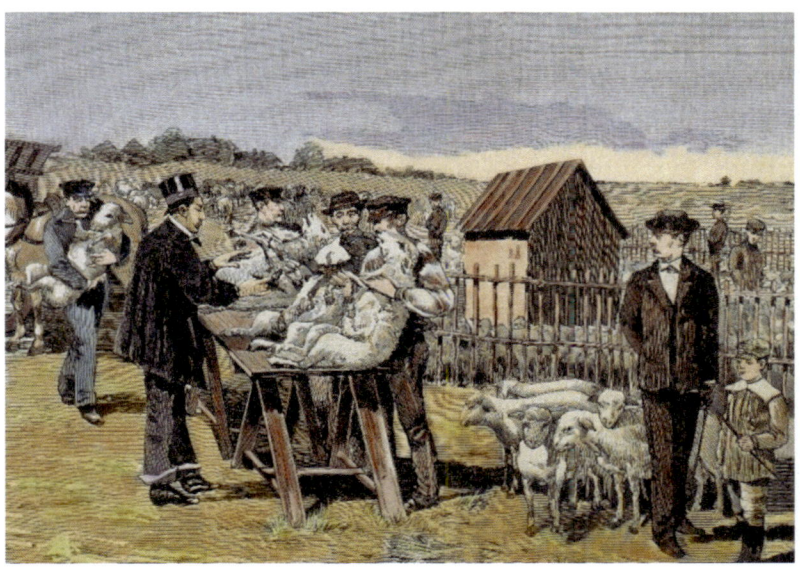

Pasteur inoculating sheep in the French villages

The publicity was intense. A reporter from the London Times sent back daily dispatches. Newspapers in France followed the events with daily bulletins. There were crowds of onlookers, farmers, engineers, veterinarians, physicians, scientists, and a carnival atmosphere. Would Pasteur's claims of vaccination hold up? Even Pasteur was privately concerned that he had acted impetuously in accepting the challenge. Happily, the trial was a complete success indeed, a triumph! Two days after final inoculation (May 5, 1882), every one of 25-control sheep was dead and every one of the 25 vaccinated sheep was alive and healthy. The fame of Pasteur and these experiments spread throughout France, Europe and beyond. It was, says Duclaux, "The anthrax vaccine that spread through the public mind faith in the science of microbes." Within 10 years, a total of 3.5 million sheep and a half-million cattle had been vaccinated with a mortality of less than 1 percent. The immediate savings to the French economy were enormous, at least seven million francs, estimated to be enough to cover the reparations that France was required to pay to Prussia for the loss of the Franco-Prussian War.

Pasteur next identified and isolated over the microbes for many other diseases including swine erysipelas, childbirth fever and pneumonia. The final and certainly most famous success of Pasteur's research was the development of a vaccine against rabies or hydrophobia as it is also known. The people of France wanted him to use it on humans, but Pasteur insisted that many years of additional research were necessary before the treatment could be tried on humans. But events made him act sooner.

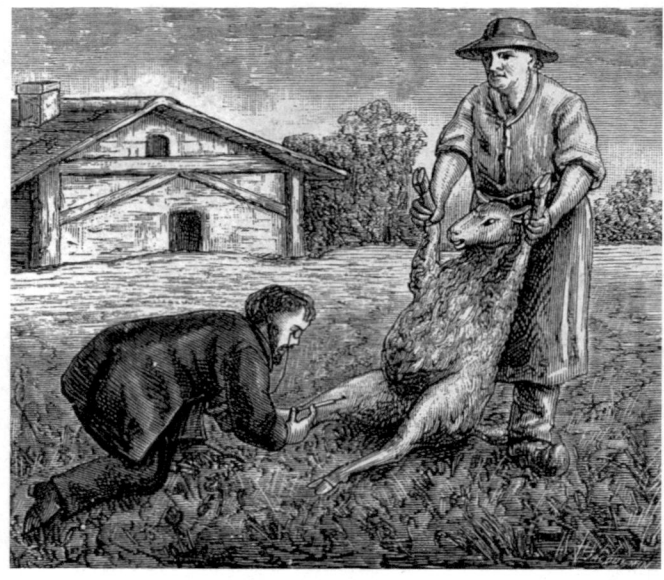

Pasteur inoculating sheep

England and Germany had long been associated by a similar language, and European royal intermarriage. Queen Victoria had married her German cousin, Prince Albert of Saxe-Coburg-Gotha and Kaiser William I's son, Prince Frederick William, just married her eldest daughter.

Bismarck, distrusted Frederick, and kept him away from politics fearing he would lead the new Empire into war as he had distinguished himself both in the Austro-Prussian War of 1866, and the Franco-Prussian War of 1870. Frederick's father, Kaiser William I, lived to the age of 91, and Frederick didn't get a chance to succeed him until late in life when he already was potentially suffering from a terminal illness. I will let Dr Lawrence I. Bonchek, is his wonderful article 'How Cancer Caused WWI and Its Aftermath' to continue the tale. The story began in January 1887 when Crown Prince Frederick complained of hoarseness, attributed to another of his frequent colds which resulted from his chain-smoking. When the Kaiser's symptoms persisted, Dr Ernst Gerhardt, a physician from Berlin, cauterized a lesion on the left vocal cord several times. When it recurred by May, eminent surgeon Dr Ernst von Bergmann was consulted, and a diagnosis of cancer was considered.

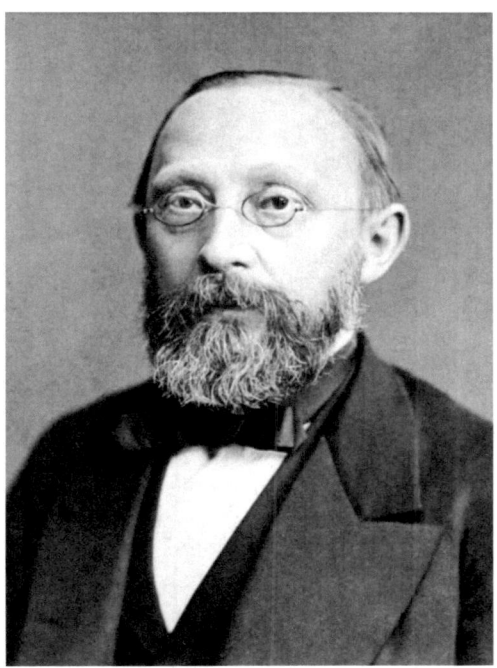

Rudolf Virchow (1821–1902). German pathologist and politician

When surgical removal was recommended, Kaiser William I and Bismarck, aware of the diagnosis, refused to subject Frederick to laryngectomy without his consent. Three other consultants advocated a more conservative approach: laryngofissure and a limited resection of one vocal cord. The lesion was early, the prince was healthy, and the surgical risk was low. Frederick would be permanently hoarse, but he would have a voice. German surgery in the late 19th Century led the world. After the introduction of ether in 1846 in America, the availability of safe and effective general anaesthesia transformed surgery. Many German surgeons gained international reputations, including Theodore Billroth, (the father of abdominal surgery) and Theodore Kocher, was awarded the Nobel Prize in 1909 for his work on the thyroid gland. Pasteur provided its scientific basis of antisepsis. The German Royal family had access to the finest surgical care in the world, and while German consultants agreed with the suspicion of malignancy, another opinion was sought from English laryngologist, Dr Morrell Mackenzie, who had published a few papers on diseases of the throat.

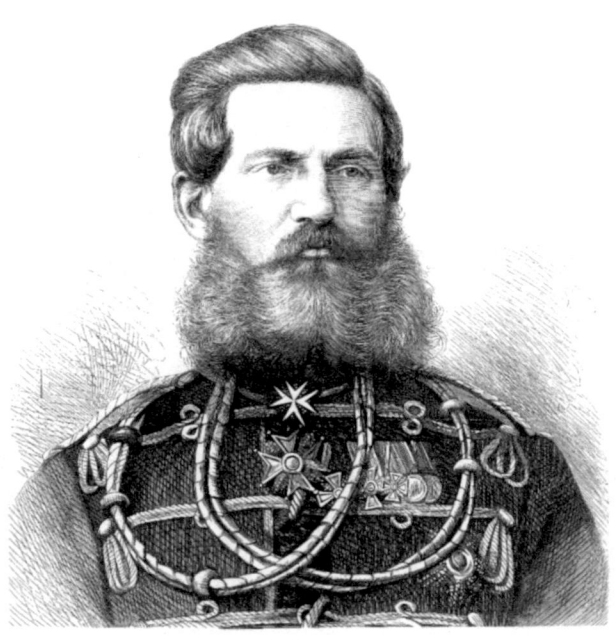

Prince William 111

Mackenzie went to Berlin and attempted a biopsy which yielded a small fragment of tissue. This was examined by Rudolf Virchow, the father of cellular pathology who saw no malignancy. Mackenzie, relying on Virchow's opinion, disagreed with the German doctor's that surgery should be done. The choice was left to Frederick, whose decision was based on emotion. Could only be based on emotion, and he decided to go with Mackenzie's diagnosis.

In fact, he attended Queen Victoria's Golden Jubilee celebration on June 21, 1887, and while there Mackenzie removed all the tumour he could find, and again Virchow failed to find evidence of a malignancy. The growth progressed nonetheless, and by autumn Frederick had completely lost his voice. When Mackenzie examined him again in November, the diagnosis and prognosis were undeniable, and Frederick was told that his life expectancy was limited. Frederick died on June 15, 1888 after only 99 days as Kaiser, during which the German public and press trashed his English wife and his English doctor for what had befallen their deservedly beloved 'Fritz'. It was the same year a great blizzard fell along the eastern seaboard of the United States, killing more than 400, and De Beers Consolidated Mines Ltd. was founded in Kimberley, South Africa. To add to the international embarrassment, Queen Victoria knighted Mackenzie for his care of her son-in-law. Mackenzie suggested that the lesion had become cancerous as a result of the treatment rendered by the German physicians after his visit to Berlin. He became ostracized because his account was so conspicuously offensive and narcissistic, and he was censured by the Royal College of Surgeons. He died suddenly at a young age in 1892, the same year that Ellis Island began receiving immigrants to the United States.

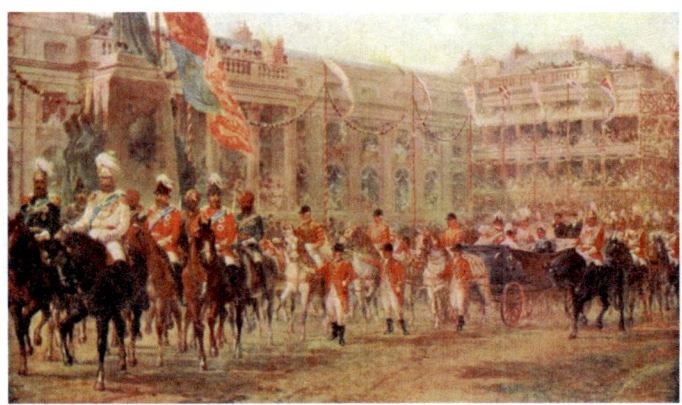

Queen Victoria's Golden jubilee, en route to Westminster Abbey, 21 June 1887

The brief reign of Kaiser Frederick III was succeeded by that of his 29-year-old eldest son William II, whose personality was profoundly influenced by an injury to his left brachial plexus at birth, which left him with a shortened, almost useless left arm. William II concealed his deformity in specially tailored uniforms and clever positioning, but he became overly sensitive to criticism and compensated by becoming volatile and aggressive. He fell out with his English mother, after the death of his father. From this period, he began building up his army and navy to challenge England's position as a world leader. He sent Bismarck into retirement and openly challenged British naval supremacy, and revised who were its allies, to suppress its historical enemy France with whom it had been at war earlier in the century. Meanwhile, Koch's colleagues at the Institute for Infectious Diseases, von Behring, Ehrlich and Kitasato, published their epoch-making work on the immunology of diphtheria. In 1896, Koch went to South Africa to study the origin of rinderpest and although he did not identify the cause of this disease, he succeeded in limiting the outbreak. He did this by injecting bile from the gall bladders of infected animals into healthy farm-stock. He also went to work in India and Africa, trying to identify the causes of malaria, blackwater fever and surra. Soon after his return to Germany, he was sent to Italy and the tropics where he confirmed the work of Sir Ronald Ross in malaria and did useful work on the aetiology of the different forms of malaria and their control with quinine.

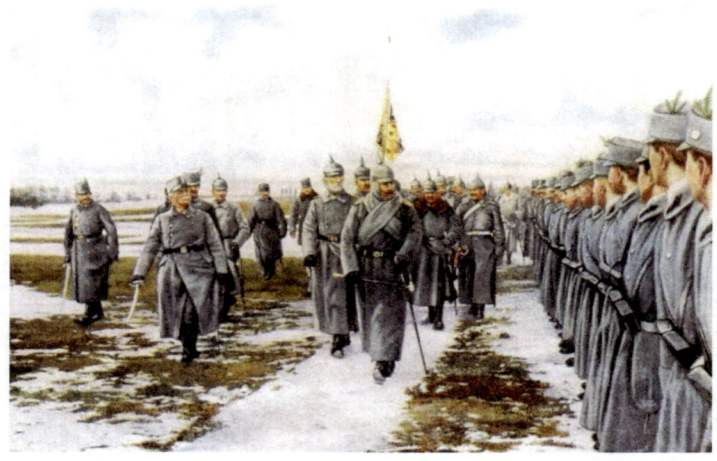

Kaiser Wilhelm (William) II, German emperor, inspects Austro-Hungarian troops on the East Galician front, New Year's Day, 1916.

But where am I with the Bacillus Anthracis story? We were recalling my exploits during the fifth plague of Egypt! (Exodus 9:3) in Egypt if I remember. Meanwhile, it was nearing the end of the reign of Queen Victoria and France and Napoleon was planning an expedition to the headwaters of the Nile that could stoke the old hostilities with England and Germany. As mentioned, Germany and England had bonds of language, culture, and shared history of wars against France. But Germany's relentless naval expansion under the new Prince led to pressure on England and forced it to realise that Germany was determined to contest England's dominance. As the new century dawned, I started spreading the good word amongst the factories, especially to the mill workers who handled infected animal hairs, wools, or hides and they called the condition 'wool sorters' or even ragpickers' disease. In the early 1900s, over a hundred people in the United States alone contracted me every year.

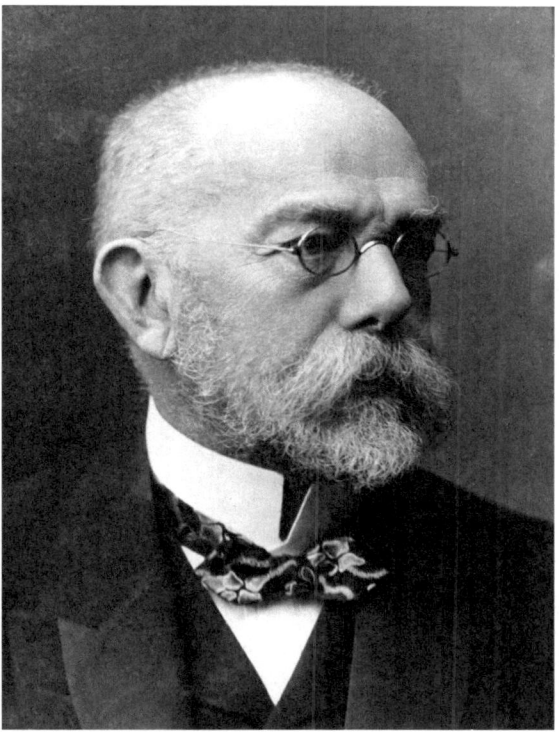

Robert Koch

Then came the First World War and I befriended Anton Dilger, an Imperial German agent who decided to grow me in a corner of his Washington home. He got his friends on the docks in Baltimore to inject my spores into over 3,000 horses and mules destined for the Allied forces in Europe. Most of the animals died, and many hundreds of soldiers on the Western Front were infected with disease. Overnight, I had become a bioweapon. The mistakes of Mackenzie and Virchow would be paid for in blood by legions of Ulstermen on the battlefields of Ypres and the Somme. By Armistice Day more than four years later on November 11, 1918, more than 9 million soldiers and an equal number of civilians had been killed, and an estimated 21 million people had been injured. Well, the years passed and in 1937, the Japanese decided to try me out again, as a bioweapon on an extended holiday in Manchuria.

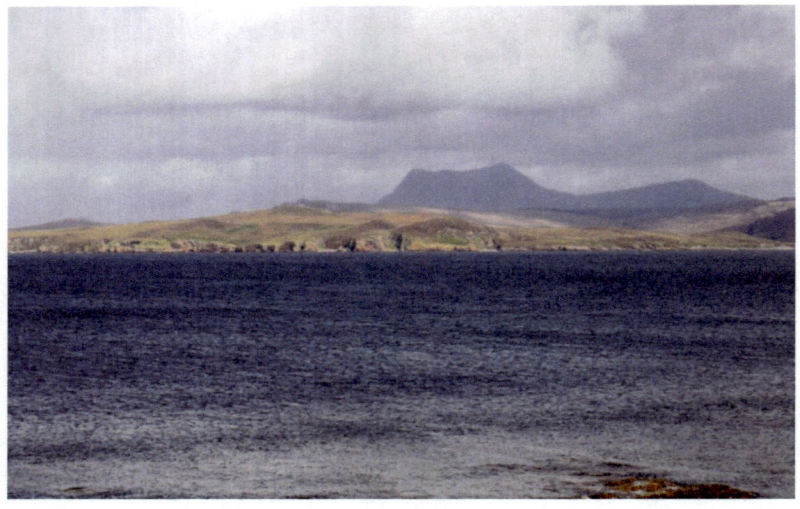

Aultbea United Kingdom Scotland GB Gruinard Island in Gruinard Bay Island where Anthrax was released during WW2

In 1942, the British military began experimenting with me on Gruinard Island, a 500-acre dot of land off the north-western coast of Scotland. They thought that I would quickly die or blow away into the ocean. But I lived on and remained infectious year after year. Finally, in 1986, after critics labelled Gruinard 'Anthrax Island', the British government decided to clean up the mess. In the spring of 1979, I killed 66 people in the industrial city of Sverdlovsk (now Yekaterinburg), Russia. In 1992, another team of Russian and U.S. scientists concluded that a local military facility had accidentally released me as a cloud, killing scores of people and animals who inhaled it. The outbreak might have provided a wealth of data about me, but true to form, the KGB confiscated most relevant medical records, leaving only autopsy notes and tissue samples behind.

Let's now head south to the world of Saddam Hussein in Iraq, who started researching me at the Muthanna chemical weapons centre in 1985. They later grew me in larger scale fermenters at their Al Salman plant, and even went into larger-scale production at Al Hakam in 1989. Saddam had manufactured over 8,500 litres by 1990 and it is generally thought that he probably wanted to send it all back by Scud missile to the land of Canaan. I mean what it is about these friends of the Pharaoh who spend half of their lives trying to get me to settle in Israel.

Then in July 1993, Aum Shinrikyo, Japan's Supreme Truth doomsday cult founded by Shoko Asahara in 1984, sprayed me as a large amount of liquid from a cooling tower on the roof of their Tokyo headquarters in 1995. The group initially started as a spiritual organization blending elements of Hindu and Buddhist beliefs. Over time, it evolved into a highly secretive and extremist group with a focus on developing and stockpiling chemical and biological weapons. In this attack, members of the cult released the deadly nerve agent sarin in the Tokyo subway system, resulting in the deaths of thirteen people and injuring thousands. The actions of Aum Shinrikyo shocked the world and brought attention to the dangers of religious extremism and terrorism. In the aftermath of the attacks, Japanese authorities cracked down on the cult, leading to the arrest and prosecution of its leaders and members. Shoko Asahara, the founder, was eventually convicted and executed in 2018.

However, their plan to use me to cause an epidemic failed. The attack resulted in a large number of complaints about bad odours but no infections. When they released the family from the building, they just couldn't hack it in the big smoke. Well, what do you expect from a crowd of frightened hillbillies that were once used as a vaccine for cattle in a Northern Arizona University? But be mindful of those Aum Shinrikyo cult members as they carried out the deadly Tokyo subway sarin attack in 1995 and were found to have been responsible for the Matsumoto sarin attack the previous year. Be careful also, because the last I saw of them, they were going to Zaire, on supposed medical mission. The actual purpose of the trip to Central Africa was to bring back samples of Ebola virus, which has since had a vaccine against it.

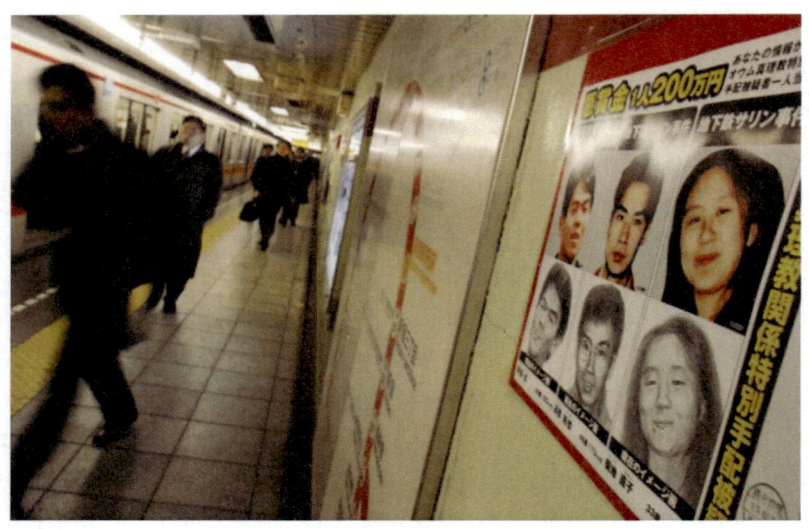

Police 'wanted' poster for members of Aum Shinrikyo Supreme Truth Cult, in Tokyo

****

Anthrax spores can exist for hundreds of years and become reactivated again. The ability of anthrax spores to endure for such extended periods is attributed to their unique structure and protective mechanisms. The spores are formed by the bacteria and allow them to withstand adverse conditions and remain viable over long periods until they encounter suitable conditions for germination and growth. It is estimated that there are around 1.5 million anthrax-infected reindeer carcasses in the arctic permafrost, and the spores can survive in the permafrost for over a hundred years. In 2016, an anthrax outbreak in reindeer was linked to a 75-year-old carcass that defrosted during global warming in the artic, and a child died in Siberia.

I am *Yersinia Pestis*, Who Caused the Plague of Justinian and the Emergence of Christianity

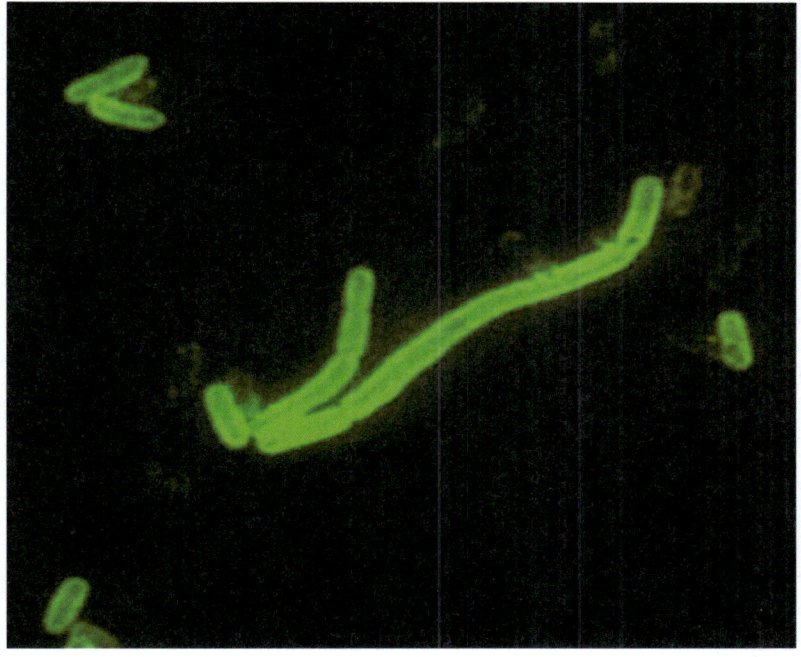

Plague bacillus Yersinia pestis, Direct Fluorescent Antibody Stain (DFA)

Yersinia pestis is a gram-negative, non-motile bacterium of the coccobacillus shape. It is the causative agent of the plague, a severe infectious disease that has had significant historical impacts. Yersinia pestis is closely related to other bacteria in the Yersinia genus, including Yersinia pseudotuberculosis and Yersinia enterocolitica. The bacterium Yersinia pestis is primarily transmitted through fleas that infest rodents, such as rats. Humans can become infected with

Yersinia pestis through flea bites or through direct contact with bodily fluids or tissues of infected animals. The plague can manifest in different forms, including bubonic, septicaemic, and pneumonic plague, each with distinct symptoms and clinical presentations. Historically, the plague caused devastating pandemics such as the Black Death in the 14th century, which resulted in millions of deaths across Europe. There may be evidence suggesting the bacterium pestis originated in Europe in the Cucuteni–Trypillia culture and not in Asia as is more commonly believed. Today, the plague is rare but still present in certain regions of the world, particularly in rural areas with limited healthcare infrastructure.

It can infect humans via the Oriental rat flea (Xenopsylla cheopis). It causes the disease plague, which takes three main forms: pneumonic, septicaemic, and bubonic.

The Plague of Justinian or Justinianic Plague (541–549 AD) was the beginning of the first plague pandemic, the first Old World pandemic of plague, the contagious disease caused by the bacterium Yersinia pestis. The disease first appeared in Egypt, and spread through Palestine, Byzantine Empire, and then throughout the Mediterranean, severely affecting both the Sasanian and the Roman Empire, most especially its capital, Constantinople. The plague changed the course of the Roman Empire, especially Emperor Justinian's plans to bring it back together and is credited with creating an apocalyptic atmosphere that spurred the rapid spread of Christianity.

This is my story.

All that great learning of Galen and Hippocrates, those physicians that taught that disease was caused by pathogenic agents was laid to waste during my reign of terror and the early Christian Church eagerly rushed to fill the medical void, becoming a doctor to body and soul, and consequently held up the advancement of medical science until probably late in the seventeenth century. The Church, in its new role as healer, equated disease with vice and sin, the punishment for people leading an errant life and not listening to the voice of Rome. Their writers, whose literary plague model was the Book of Revelation, promoted and prolonged this idea. There was John of Ephesus who clearly said that the end of the world was at hand, or Zachariah of Mytilene who said that the plague was a scourge from Satan and even the more reasonable Gregory of Tours said people could only be saved by praying to St Gall. Well, add in a few wonders like the collapse of the original dome of Hagia Sophia during the earthquake of

Constantinople and its little wonder that the religiosity of the Byzantine Empire dramatically increased during this period. It was like the twin towers falling without a valid reason. Anyway, to get back to poor Justinian after whom I am so nobly called. Let me tell you a little about him. In his day, he was also known as Flavius Petrus Sabbatius Justinianus, the great Byzantine Emperor whose architectural monuments still lie strewn around Istanbul and beyond. Thank God, they didn't call me after his real name. In 525, at the age of 42, he received the title of Caesar and two years later the rank of Augustus. It was a time of great splendour as Justinian erected magnificent buildings, recruited armies and formed codes of laws, which became the basis of European Justice.

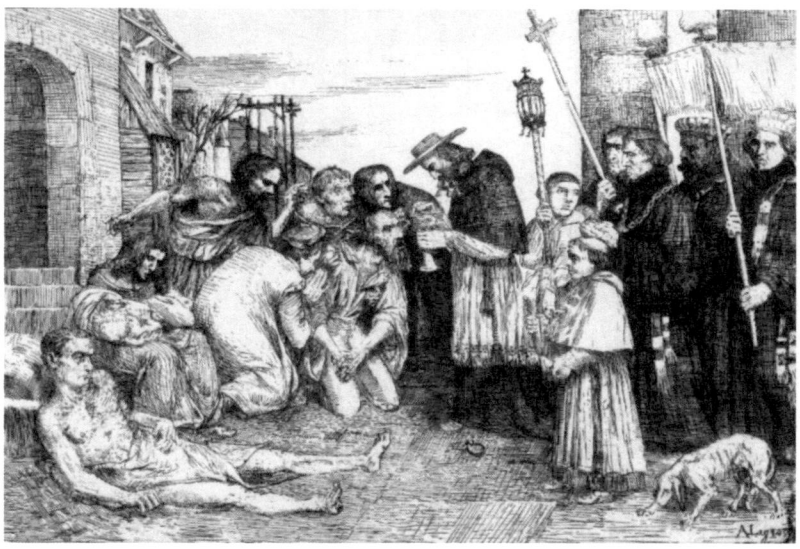

The Plague of Justinian

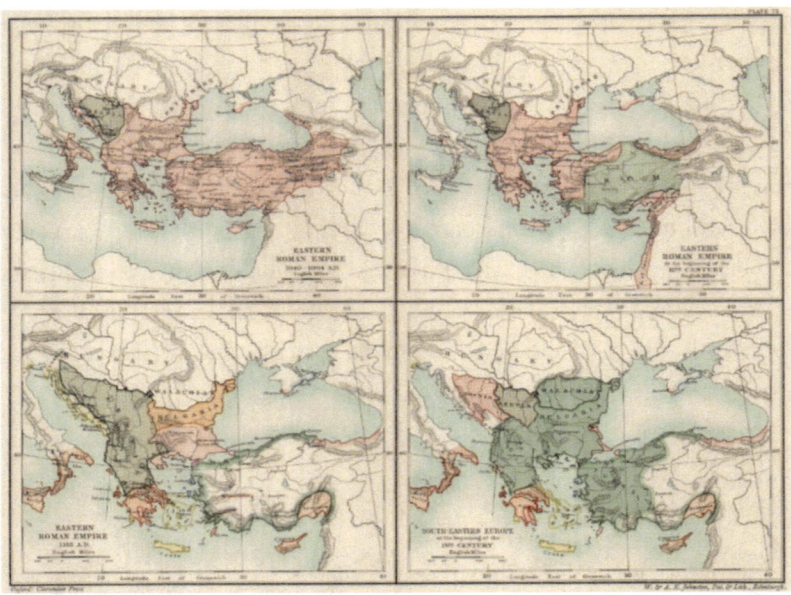

Eastern Roman/Byzantine Empire: 1040–1064; 1100; 1355

People followed the teachings of progressive physicians who were creating the discipline of medical science. Into this noble world, I came wreaking destruction and forming the worst pandemic that has harrowed human kind. Today, the record of my destruction remains amongst three main sources, John of Ephesus, who wrote Historia Ecclesiastica, while wandering around the empire, the lesser known Evagrius Scholasticus and last but not least, Justinian's archivist, Procopius, who published the History of the Wars, in 550.

I started my long march around the Empire in 540. In that year, I befriended people in Pelsium, Lower Egypt and within a month traders and itinerant scholars had carried me to Alexandria and Palestine. Now I won't argue with Procopius when he said that the death toll in Constantinople, in spring of 542 became 10,000 a day, but allowing for a small exaggeration, this was more people than Justinian was losing in his battles against Italy and Persia. At any rate, following my sojourn in Constantinople, I spread throughout the empire along with trade and military routes from the coastal cities to the interior provinces. I surfaced in Italy in 543, and from there, migrated to Persia, to infect the Persian army and King Khusro himself, causing them to retreat east of the Tigris to the plague-free highlands of Luristan.

Gregory of Tours tells how St Gall saved the people of Clermont-Ferrand in Gaul from me in 543, and I visited Ireland for a short period in 544. I left as the barmen told me Guinness wouldn't be around for another 1225 years. At least, they couldn't blame the Black Stuff on the Dubliners that were breaking out in black blisters, vomiting blood and some others seized by madness. And the poor doctors, not knowing what to do, just lanced the buboes and looked at the withered thighs and tongues and hoped they were living in 1784, when a few of the lads from the newly opened Royal College of Surgeons could help them in their work. But these were other days, when in typical apocalyptic literature style, John of Ephesus seen hallucinations as 'apparitions' from another worldly realm, when men wore identification tags with the fear of being left unburied and ships floated aimlessly at sea, later washing up to shore with all of their crew having become my friends Although the emperor Justinian contracted the disease himself, he valiantly attempted to minimise the disaster. Following the outbreak in Constantinople, Justinian commanded the palace guard to dispose of the corpses. But soon all the gravesites were filled beyond capacity, and the living resorted to throwing the bodies of victims out into the streets or piling them along the seashore to rot. He responded to this problem by having huge pits dug across the Golden Horn in Sycae and hiring men to collect the dead. Although these pits reportedly held 70,000 corpses each, they soon overflowed, and Justinian ordered that the bodies should be placed inside the towers of the city walls and to pour lime down the shafts. When the decaying corpses caused a stench that pervaded the entire city, he ordered that the rotting dead should be put on ships and set fire at sea. Procopius also recorded the human dimension of the tragedy. The first day the person could feel the hard nodes or 'buboes' in the armpits and groin. By the second and third day, the fever produced violent delirium in which the victims hallucinated, seeing 'phantoms of death'.

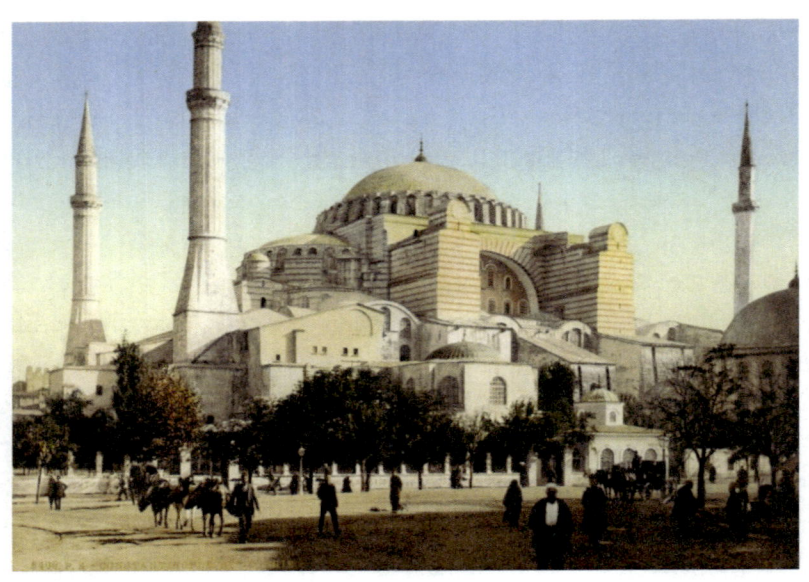

Hagio Sophia, Constantinople exterior view, built by Anthemius of Tralles and Isidore of Miletus from 532–537

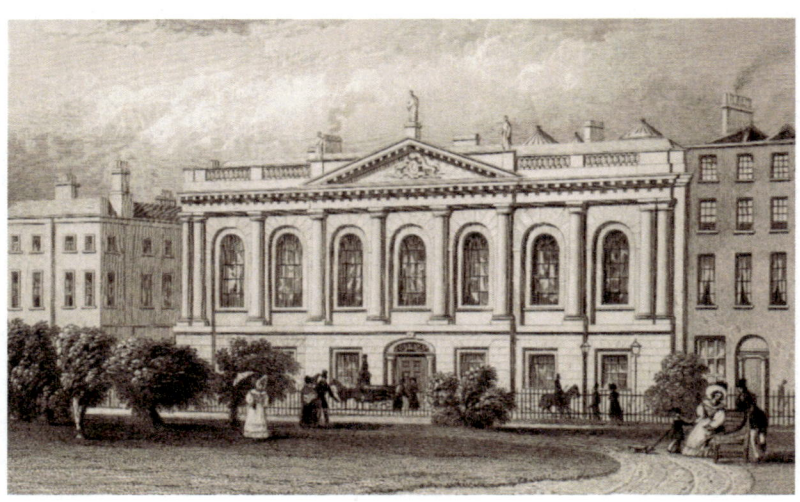

Royal College of Surgeons, Dublin

He astutely observed that a person who coughed and spit up phlegm died quickly, usually by the fifth day. Students from the Royal College of Surgeons today, God bless 'em, would tell you that I actually came in three forms: bubonic, pneumonic (also called pulmonary), and the septicaemic.

The bubonic form, which must exist before the other two strains can become active, is not directly contagious unless the patient harbours fleas. Since Procopius did not state that those who cared for the sick necessarily contracted the disease, it is inferred that the bubonic form was most active in the Justinianic plague. The pneumonic plague occurred whenever I decided to invade the lungs. This variety is highly contagious from one person to another and is spread by airborne droplets. Due to Procopius' observation that the plague was not directly contagious, and the absence of the major symptoms of pneumonic plague in the accounts, namely shallow breathing and tightness in the chest, this form was probably not highly active. Septicaemia occurs when the infection enters the bloodstream, and death is swift, usually before buboes are able to form. In his account, Agathias reported some of my friends dying as if by an attack of apoplexy and from this some scholars would deduct that my septicaemic form did exist during the Justinian outbreak. But either way, I wreak disaster as bubonic plague results in 70% deaths; pneumonic plague in 90% and septicaemic plague leaves no survivors. To live for ten days was considered a miracle and gave time for one to offer additional prayers for an inevitable end.

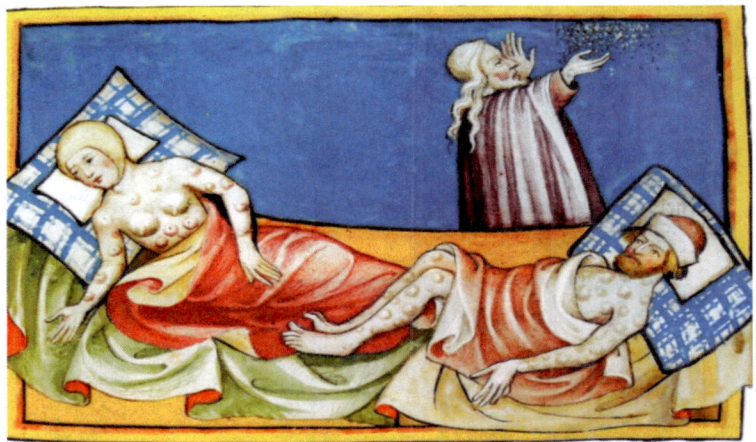

Miniature out of the Toggenburg Bible (Switzerland) of 1411. The disease is widely believed to be the plague. The location of bumps or blisters, however, is more consistent with smallpox (as the bubonic plague normally causes them only in the groin and in the armpits). Is generally interpreted as a depiction of the plague—'the Black Death'.

It was common for entire families and professions to be wiped out, their lineage ended and their professions to be lost to history. During the half century that the Justinian plague raged, no village or town was spared, and one hundred million people died of the disease. This meant that recruits for the Roman Army became difficult to find, with the result that the empire was mostly served by barbarian mercenaries. In Justinian's final years, there were virtually no men either to volunteer or to be impressed into the service. Because he was spared, he withdrew from public life and devoted himself to theological problems. He believed that Christ was entirely divine and that his incorruptible human body was just a delusion. This blasphemy didn't suit the Christians of the period and nobody was surprised when he died two years later. Fortunately for the Romans themselves, the plague had also attacked and weakened the Persian Empire. In Italy, the Ostrogoths resumed the war, and new revolts broke out in the previously subdued African provinces. Needless to say, the Justinianic plague, apart from its devastating immediate impact, undermined the political and economic structure of the late Roman Empire, creating conditions ripe for disaster. Coupled with the other disasters, the plague reduced the population of the Mediterranean world by 40% by the year 600. Such a massive mortality rate caused depopulation of the urban centres and created a structural imbalance in favour of the desert Arabs. But before I go down that road, let us just say that I was a microbe that changed the history of the world!

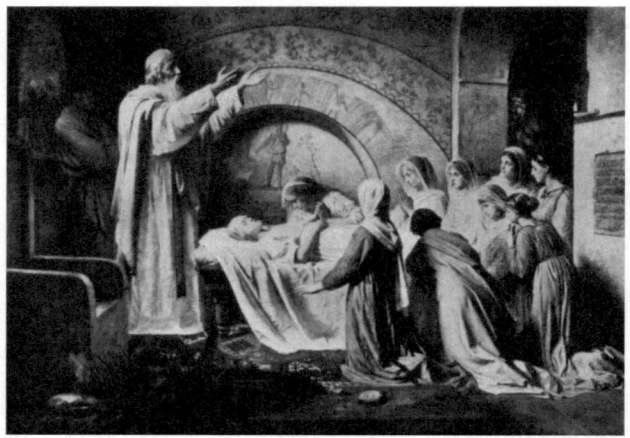

Historicizing representation of a funeral in the catacombs of Rome, the underground burial places of the early Christians in ancient Rome. After a painting by A. Grass from around 1890.

Description from the handbook of medical entomology. The record of its ravages is almost beyond belief. In 542 AD, it caused ten thousand deaths in Constantinople in one day. In the 14th century, it spread from the East throughout Armenia, Asia Minor, Egypt, Northern Africa, and Europe. Hecker estimates that one-fourth of the population of Europe, or twenty-five million persons, died in the epidemic of that century. From then until the 17th century, it was almost constantly present in Europe, including the great plague of London, in 1665 killing 68,596 out of the population. Recurrences over the next two centuries eventually killed about 50 million people, 26 percent of the world population. It is believed to be the first significant appearance of the bubonic plague, which features enlarged lymphatic gland and is carried by rats and spread by fleas. Based upon DNA analysis of bones found in graves, the type of plague that struck the Byzantine Empire during the reign of Justinian was bubonic (Yersinia pestis), although it was very probable that the other two types of plague, pneumonic and septicaemic, were also present.

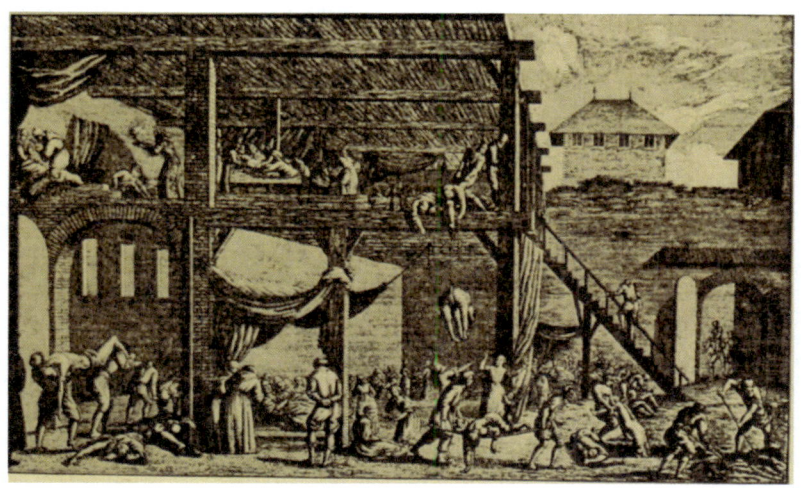

Deaths in Constantinople 542 AD

Plague has a complicated cause involving a pathogen, originally named *Pasteurella pestis*, but now universally termed *Yersinia pestis*. This oval bacterium was discovered simultaneously in 1894 in Hong Kong by Alexandre Yersin, a Swiss student of Louis Pasteur, and by the Japanese physician Shibasaburo Kitasato, a protégé of Pasteur's rival Robert Koch. also known as the Plague of Galen (after Galen, the Greek physician who described it).

160 A.D.: Antonian Plague was brought to the Roman Empire by troops who were returning from campaigns in the Middle East. Most historians agree that the plague appeared first during the Roman siege of Seleucia, a major Mesopotamian city of the Seleucid, Parthian, and Sasanian empires, which stood on the west bank of the Tigris River near present-day Baghdad in Iraq. Scholars have suspected it to have been either smallpox or measles. The plague broke out again nine years later in 189 AD and caused up to 2,000 deaths a day in Rome, with a mortality rate of nearly 30%. The total death count has been estimated to be about 5–10 million, and the disease killed as much as one third of the population and devastated the Roman army.

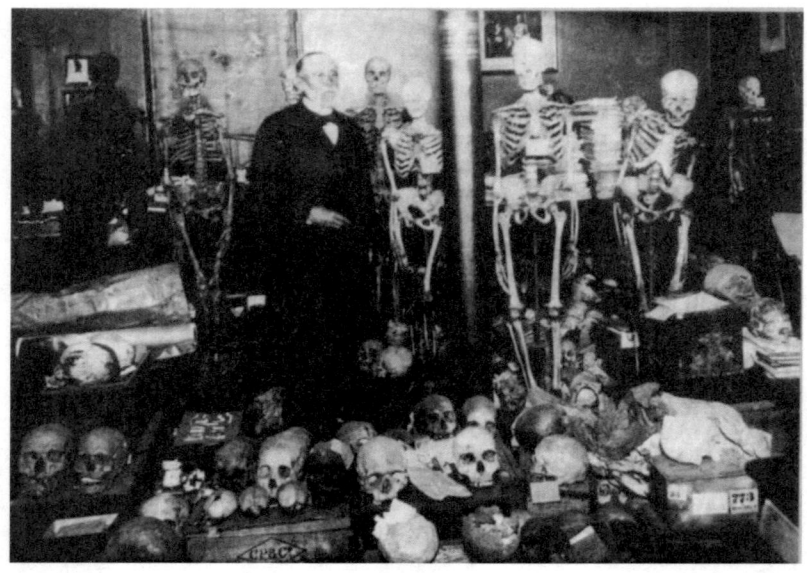

Virchow in his pathology laboratory

250 A.D.: Cyprian Plague presented and was named after the first known victim, the Christian bishop of Carthage, the Cyprian plague victims exhibited a fever, vomiting, diarrhoea, throat ulcers, and gangrenous hands and feet. It was largely spread by a urban to rural transmigration as people tried to escape becoming a victim. It began in Africa and spread to Rome, Greece and back to Egypt.

444 A.D: British Plague Again, it recurred and changed the course of history with recurring outbreaks over the next three centuries. In 444 A.D., it hit Britain and obstructed defence efforts against the Picts and the Scots, causing the British to seek help from the Saxons, who would soon control the island. It ravaged Britain over the next hundred years, causing many deaths. Scientists have recently discovered genetic material from buried mummies who died of the plague in Cambridgeshire in 544 AD.

The number of deaths relating to the Justinian Plague remains uncertain, but probably around thirty million people. Some historians believe that the plague killed up to 5,000 people per day in Constantinople at the peak of the pandemic, wiping out perhaps 40% of the city's inhabitants and caused the deaths a lot of the population of the Eastern Mediterranean. Others that the plague might have caused high mortality in specific places, but it did not cause widespread demographic decline or decimate Mediterranean populations. There is no doubt that later waves of the plague saw the disease becoming more localised and less virulent.

I Am *Yersinia Pestis*, Who Caused Typhus, the Emergence of Protestantism, and the Destruction of Napoleon's 'Grande Armee'

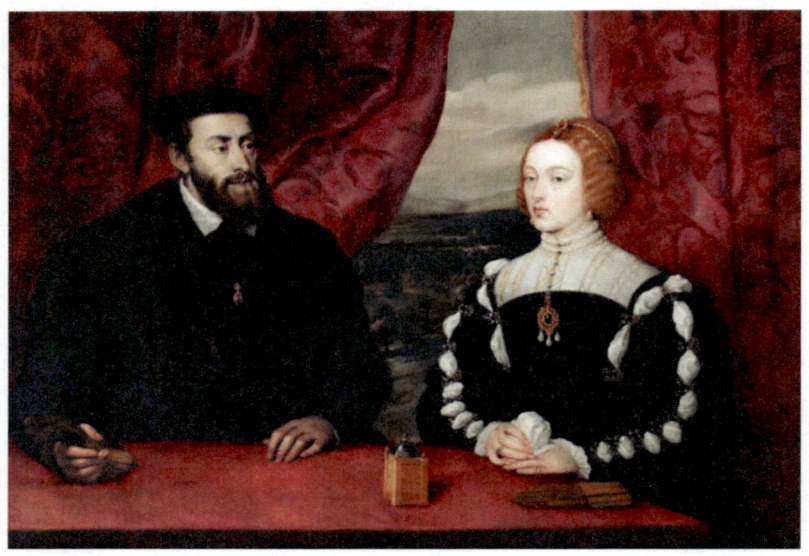

Charles V and Empress Isabella of Portugal-Titian

In the early part of the Sixteenth Century, both the French and Spanish were locked in a struggle to determine which was to be the major power and controlling force in Europe. Even though both countries were Catholic and comparable military strength, I played a large role in determining the rise of the Protestant religion in Europe. It all began whenever Pope Clement VII decided to secretly favour Francis I of France because of a debt owed to him by the King of Italy, although protocol demanded that he show no outward preference. So, in 1525, the Pope advised Francis I to march into Italy and gain control over the papal states. However, this became a terrible misadventure as he was ambushed by the large Spanish army of Charles V and taken prisoner. The Spanish finding out about the Pope's favouritism then turned towards Rome, forcing Pope Clement VII to flee the Vatican. The Spanish burned Rome inciting the anger of other Christian European nations, especially as the Muslim Ottoman Turks were threatening to invade Italy from the east.

At this time, an epidemic of Plague struck the Spanish within the city of Naples and reduced their diseased army to 11,000. The French finally arrived and laid siege to the city but then I arrived and within a month, 25,000 French soldiers perished of the disease. All of Europe looked upon the deadly pestilence that obliterated the French army as an act of God. Their downfall resulted in Charles V being crowned Holy Roman Emperor in 1530. The Church played along with the belief that God created epidemics to get rid of sinners and they opposed the science that tried to understand them. Now that he was Holy Roman Emperor, his army went to Metz, Germany to subdue the rising ideology of Protestantism in Northern Europe. Because of my interference, ten thousand of his troops died from typhus in the first month of siege. As a result, he was never able subdue the rise of Protestantism. It is quite amazing that people would believe that God favoured one side of the War and when they were obliterated, he would then wipe out the other. Surely, someone could see that it was a contagious disease rather than a vengeful God at work. Charles V as Holy Emperor favoured Maximillian II, from Austria-Hungary in the thirty years' war, and protected Christian Europe from the constant wars against the Ottoman Turks, threatening to invade Europe from the East. In 1560, the Turks invaded Christian Hungary, but I caused typhus in the Austrian Hungarian troops, killing 30,000 troops, leaving Hungary in Turkish hands. Maximillian II responded by mobilizing a great Christian army and marching on the invaders, driving them out of Hungary but again they were struck down by typhus, and they had to return before finally driving the Saracens back to Turkey. In the same period, we had great physicists like Albert Einstein, Max Planck, and Wilhelm Rontgen, so don't ever say I didn't contribute something to this world.

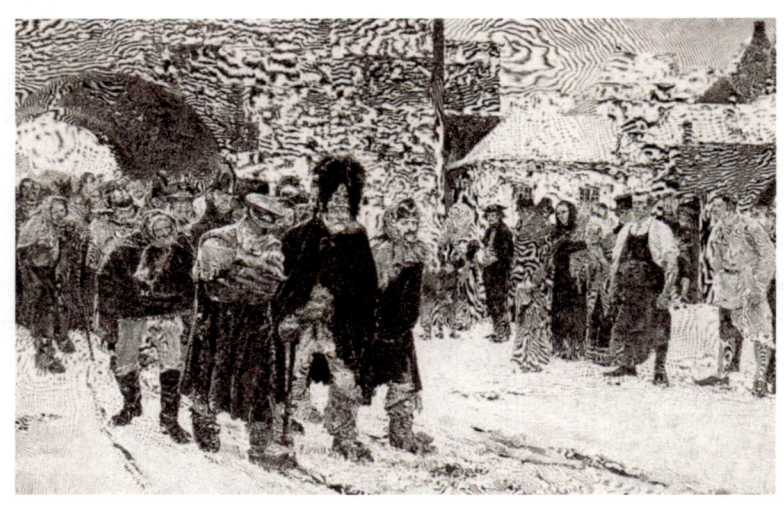

Retreat of Napoleon's remaining Grande Armée, 1812, Russian Campaign

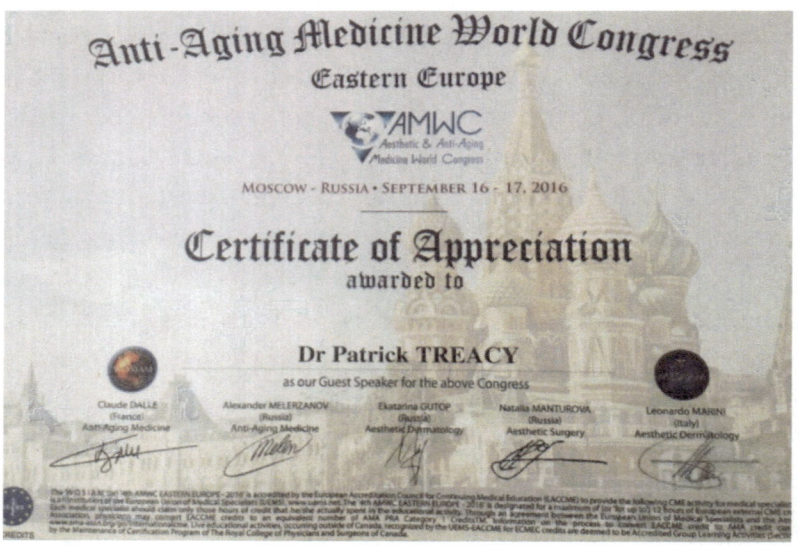

The author awarded a certificate of appreciation in Moscow.

Meanwhile, Napoleon Bonaparte had organised his 'Grande Armee', of 600,000 well-seasoned troops to conquer Europe, invade Russia, and then take India from the British in an attempt to restore France's former glory. In Autumn 1812, he left Germany to enter Poland to reach the Russian border. He employed a medical corps and respected sanitation. Unfortunately, Poland had large endemic foci of typhus and the peasantry were rife with disease. As a consequence, he forbade the soldiers to fraternize with the Polish citizenry under pain of death. He didn't take advice about the winter and when his army ran out of food and supplies, his soldiers started raiding the infected villages and nearly one hundred thousand of died in the first weeks of the campaign. Still, the heavily infected army marched on the Russian border in December of 1812, with the objective of capturing Moscow still its final goal. The Russian army knew the situation and didn't engage them, drawing them further and further into Russia as the winter worsened. They just sent in raiding parties to kill the frostbitten typhus-infected soldiers of the 'Grande Armee'. The morale of Napoleon's soldiers sank, and typhus started killing more. Amazingly, they captured Moscow in January of 1813 with only 90,000 left out of the original army of 600,000. I had killed as many as a third of a million of his men. When they entered Moscow, they found that all the food stores had been burned by the Russians and realising the war had been lost, Napoleon made for a full-scale retreat back to France. Epidemic Typhus and frostbite continued to take their toll-the portion of Napoleon's Grand Armee of 600,000 that finally reached France numbered only 20,000. Of these, only 3,000 remained alive by June of 1813.

I Am Mycobacterium Leprae, the Cause of Leprosy, and so Much Misery Worldwide

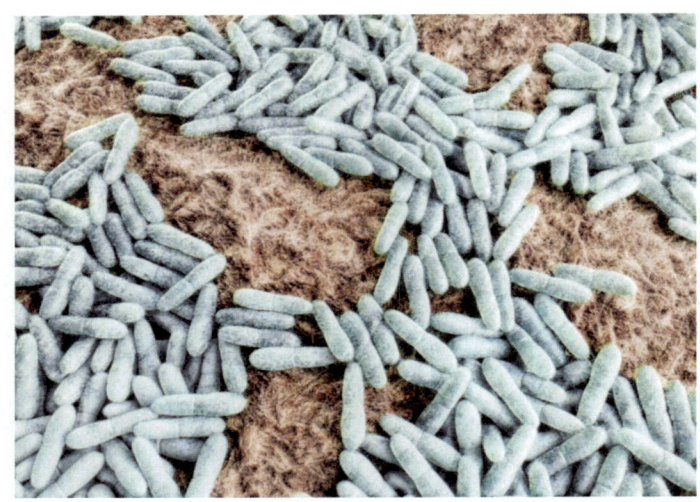

Illustration of Mycobacterium leprae, a gram-positive bacterium which is the cause of leprosy (Hansen's disease).

Mycobacterium leprae is a species of bacteria that causes Hansen's disease, also known as leprosy. It is one of the two bacteria species responsible for this chronic and curable infectious disease that primarily affects the skin, peripheral nerves, and respiratory tract. Leprosy is a chronic granulomatous infection generally caused by Mycobacterium leprae and Mycobacterium lepromatosis, both of which primarily affects the skin and peripheral nerves. Leprosy is characterized by the development of skin lesions, nerve damage, and impaired sensation. The disease progresses slowly and can lead to severe deformities if left untreated. Mycobacterium leprae is transmitted through respiratory droplets from infected individuals, but it is not highly contagious and requires prolonged close contact for transmission to occur. Although leprosy has been stigmatized throughout history, it is now well-understood and can be effectively treated with multi-drug therapy. Early diagnosis and treatment are crucial to prevent complications and disability associated with the disease.

It is curable with multidrug therapy. Treatment of paucibacillary leprosy is with the medications dapsone, rifampicin, and clofazimine for six months. Treatment for multibacillary leprosy uses the same medications for 12 months. Several other antibiotics may also be used.

This is my story.

Like many other pandemics, I started my life in Asia, where there is skeletal evidence of me being in India about 4,000 years ago. There is also evidence from 2000 BC, as found in human remains from Balathal in India and Harappa in Pakistan, however, it may have been a cousin of mine. Then, Hippocrates in 460 BC writes about a patient with skin afflictions and other leprosy-like symptoms. Either way, let me introduce myself, I am a mycobacterium with some heavy-hitting cousins like my uncle *mycobacterium tuberculosis*. And, if that isn't bad enough, I tend to hang around with armadillos, chimpanzees, mangabey monkeys, and cynomolgus macaque. Within the southern US, the M. leprae strain is native in the nine-banded armadillo and I am responsible for about 100 people are diagnosed with leprosy in the U.S. every year, mostly in the South, California, Hawaii, and some U.S. territories. The countries with the highest number of new leprosies diagnoses every year are India, Brazil, and Indonesia. More than half of all new cases of leprosy are diagnosed in India.

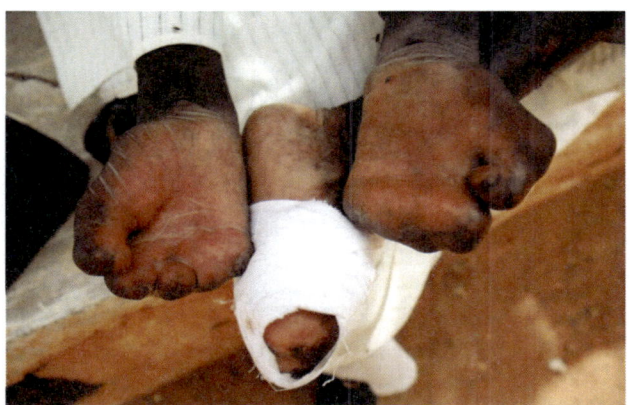

Leprosy patient known also as a Leper.

Leprosy probably did not exist in Greece or the Middle East before Common Era, which makes one wonder whether Hippocrates (c. 460–c. 370 BC), father of medicine, ever met me at all. There is some evidence to suggest leprosy also appeared in China very early, but it did not appear in the lands of Canaan or Egypt until well after Moses' time, about three centuries before Christ. In those days, those with my disease were known as 'lepers' and made to wear distinctive clothing and carry a bell or a clapper to warn people of their approach as they were social outcasts. People were so afraid of catching the disease that leper colonies on islands became widespread in the Middle Ages, particularly in Europe and India, and were often run by religious monastic orders. Historically, leprosy was feared as it caused visible disfigurement and disability, was incurable, and was commonly believed to be highly contagious. In this instance, the Catholic Church helped to run these leper colonies, which were often called lazar houses, after Lazarus, the patron saint of people affected with leprosy. I often wondered whether their benevolence in this instance, compared to their actions during cholera or syphilis was due to the fact that Jesus Christ helped Lazarus. We are reminded of the story in the bible.

"A man full of leprosy came and knelt before Him and inquired him saying, 'Lord, if you are willing, you can make me clean.' Multiple people who were lepers followed this man to get cured. 'Be clean!' Instantly he was healed of his leprosy. Then Jesus said to him, 'See that you don't tell anyone.'"

We also know, leprosy did not exist in the Americas before European colonisation nor in Polynesia until the middle of the 19th century. During the later nineteenth century, knowledge in medicine advanced tremendously. As mentioned before, this scientific period began in the late 1850s with the wonderful work of Louis Pasteur, and this was later extended by Robert Koch in the 1880s.

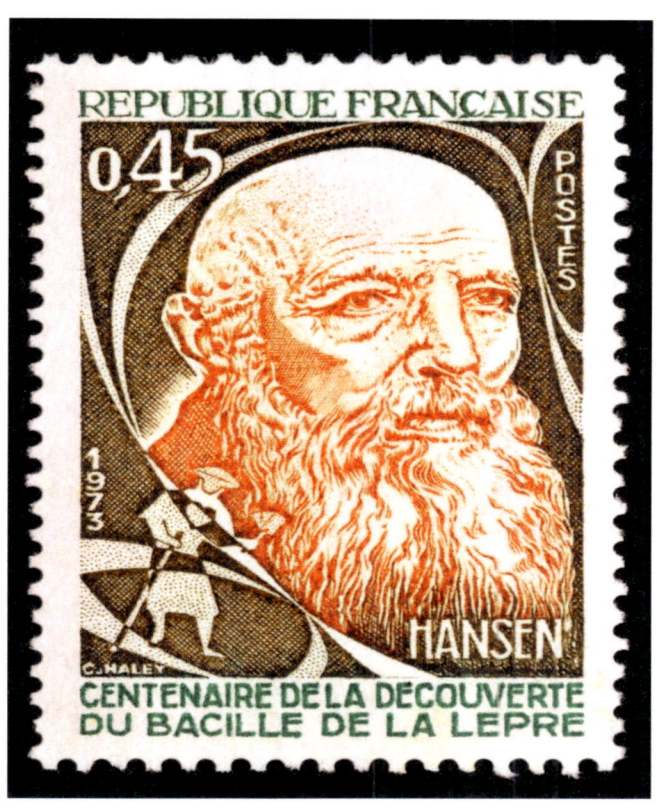

Gerhard Henrik Hansen (1841–1912). Centenary of the discovery of the leprosy / Hansen's Disease.

In 1879, a Norwegian physician called Dr Gerhard Henrik Hansen (29 July 1841–12 February 1912) was looking down a basic microscope and saw me through an inexpensive lens in the tissues of all sufferers. He called me *mycobacterium leprae,* although he did not identify myself as bacteria, and received little support from his colleagues. Hansen gave the tissue samples to Albert Neisser, who then successfully stained the bacteria and announced his findings in 1880, claiming to have discovered the disease-causing organism. Although, Hassen was the first person to identify the germ that causes leprosy under a microscope, Neisser tried to downplay his assistance. Hansen's claim was weakened by his failure to grow *mycobacterium leprae* on a culture medium, or even to prove that the rod-shaped organisms were infectious. Neisser did this and proved that leprosy was caused by a germ, and was thus not hereditary, from a curse, or from a sin. In the end, Hansen attempted to infect at least one female patient without consent and although no damage was caused, he ended up in court and lost his post at the hospital. In the end, the dispute between the two doctors was settled with Hansen being recognised as the discoverer of the bacillus and Neisser as the identifier of it being the etiological agent causing leprosy. I have a slight tendency to prefer younger people, and most of the disease develops in people aged 5 to 15 years or over 30. The incidence of leprosy peaks in two age groups (10–15 and 30–60 years of age) and there is a male predominance in most regions of about 2:1. The incubation period varies widely from months to over 30 years, but is usually prolonged, averaging four years for tuberculoid and ten years for lepromatous leprosy. Even though I appear to be highly contagious, more than 95% of people whom I infect with *mycobacterium leprae* do not develop and disease because their immune system fights off the infection. Hence, it is a myth that I am highly contagious, and the chances are you can't catch it by touching someone who has the disease. In fact, most cases of leprosy are from repeated and long-term contact with someone who has the disease. Dr Gerhard Henrik Armauer Hansen had suffered from syphilis since the 1860s but died of heart disease.

When someone gets infected, I tend to attack the nerves of the fingers and toes and cause them to become numb. This, in turn, gives rise to accidents, and burns and cuts may go unnoticed, leading to infection and permanent damage. I also cause painless ulcers, flat, pale areas of skin, and eye damage due to dryness and reduced blinking. There is no doubt that once I become established, large ulcerations, loss of digits, skin nodules, and facial disfigurement may develop. The infection spreads from person to person by nasal secretions or droplets. In the last few decades, particularly with the advent of multidrug therapy (MDT) and the use of anti-inflammatory therapies, there have been substantial improvements in long-term health outcomes for individuals diagnosed with Hansen's Disease (HD).

In 2000, the World Health Organization (WHO) identified leprosy as completely eradicated. Ultimately, infection elimination was defined as the overall reduction in prevalence to less than 1 case per 10,000 people. In the span from 1985 to 2011, the recorded cases fell from 5.4 million to approximately 219,000. By 2011, the prevalence rate in terms of 10,000 people, dropped from approximately 21.1 to 0.37, excluding Europe. Today, about 208,000 people worldwide are infected with leprosy, according to the World Health

Organization, most of them in Africa and Asia. In 2015, mortality rates fell from 4.3 to 2.5 deaths per 100,000 population. In 2018, there were 208,619 new cases of leprosy recorded, a slight decrease from 2017.

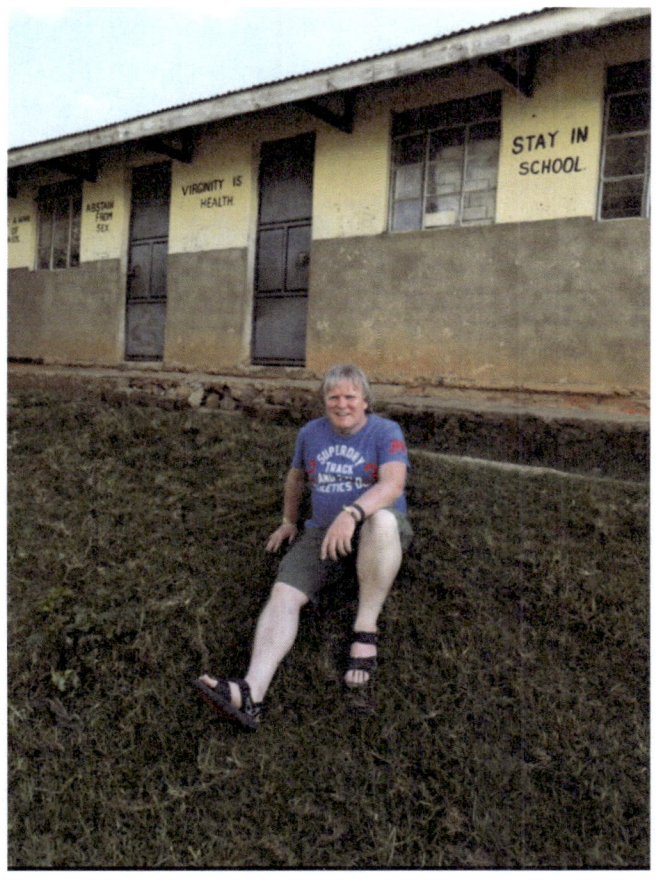

At the old leprosy school on Bwama Island, Lake Bunyonyi Uganda

I usually spend some time each year doing some humanitarian work in Africa. The African Region has the second largest prevalence of leprosy among the WHO regions with about 1 per 1,000 population affected. With a very uneven distribution among countries, the region currently has a total of about 480,000 registered cases. However, I have never seen a case there. There are memories of previous leper colonies, such as the place where Nelson Mandela's cell prison was built on Robben Island in South Africa. Leprosy broke out in the Cape during the mid-1800s, and the patients were placed out on that island. While visiting Bwama Primary School on Lake Bunyonyi in Uganda, I discovered that a British doctor and Christian missionary, Dr Leonard Sharp had been there before me. Leonard made the then uninhabited Bwama island a leper treatment and quarantine centre, back in 1931. At its height, Bwama Island had over six hundred leper patients on it, technically removing them from the communities where they might potentially infect others. The people on the island lived as a community and eventually had children, and they built Bwama Primary School in 1934 for their education. At that moment, I realised the sacrifice that some of these children must make to become educated, as every day, the Bwama Primary school's pupils had to arrive on the island in dugout canoes. Many come from other islands, but most of the pupils came from the mainland.

Risk Factors for leprosy

- Factors attributing to the contraction of leprosy include:
- Armadillo Exposure: Within the southern US, the M. leprae strain is native in the nine-banded armadillo.
- Age: Older members of society are more prone to risk in the acquisition of leprosy.
- Close Contact: Direct contact with a patient with leprosy.
- Genetic Influences: As previously mentioned, genetics plays a role in the immunologic response.
- Immunosuppression: Following the suppression of the immune system, there is an increased chance of acquiring this infection.

In 1943, Guy Faget, working at Carville Hospital in Louisiana, demonstrated that sulfone drugs were effective in killing M. leprae bacilli but despite multidrug therapy (MDT) three decades ago, the global incidence remains high. Patients also often have long-term complications associated with the disease. There is no vaccine generally available to specifically prevent leprosy, but the BCG vaccine used against my cousin, *mycobacterium tuberculosis* (TB), may provide some protection against leprosy.

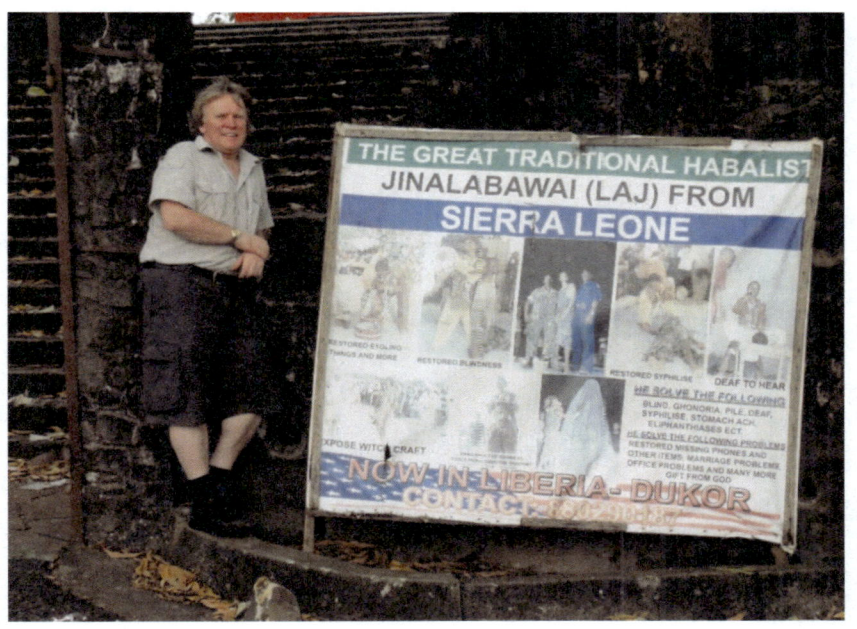

Author with sign covering all types of illness in Sierra Leone in 2012

I Am *Mycobacterium tuberculosis*, and I Was with John Keats When He Died

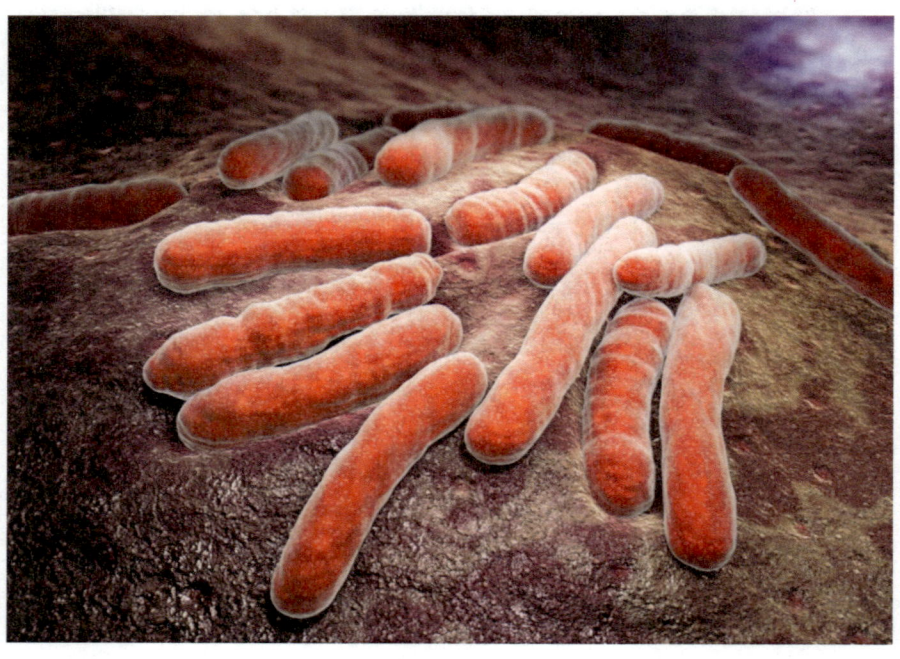

Tuberculosis (TB) is an infectious disease usually caused by Mycobacterium tuberculosis (MTB) bacteria, the causative agent of most cases of the disease. *It generally affects the lungs but can also affect other parts of the body. The classic symptoms of active TB are a chronic cough with blood-containing mucus, fever, night sweats, and weight loss. About 10% of latent infections progress to active disease which, if left untreated, kills about half of those affected. It was historically called consumption due to the weight loss.*

I am *Mycobacterium tuberculosis*, a hardy bacillus that has been on this planet so long now, that I'm actually older than the human species itself. I mean I could bore you and tell you I've seen it all, about way back in history when the green lands of Africa were still joined to Antarctica and was called Gondwanaland, but I'll not! Just suffice to say that the first recorded European consumer lived in the beautiful Altstadt of Heidelberg about seven thousand years ago. That was back in 5,000 BC, and his recently retrieved skeletal remains shows he was a true believer in the consumer cause. Around the same time, I was visiting ancient Egypt, fiddling with the dear old mummy's remains, twisting a spine here and there, sitting out on the warm hotel terrace above the Nile, hanging around waiting on the pyramid of Cheops to be built. And as the saffron sunset over the city of Cairo for the thousandth time, I legged it to India and destroyed the intricate caste system for a few thousand years.

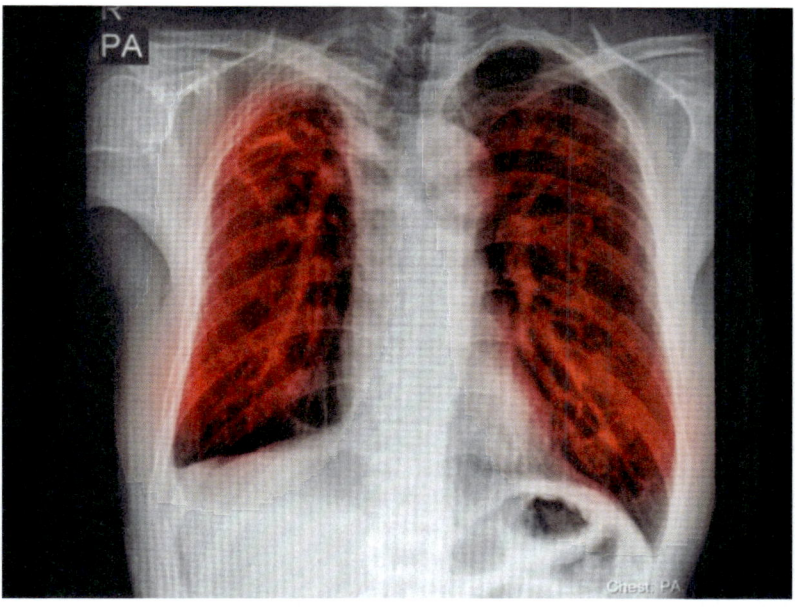

Pulmonary Tuberculosis (TB): Chest x-ray show alveolar infiltration at both lung due to mycobacterium tuberculosis infection

Then came the Greeks and Romans, good coughers one and all, except may I say that quack Hippocrates was a bit suspect, a sort of Wagnerian alter ego. I mean he actually blamed the Scandinavians for spreading the good cough about. Well, yes, I am well known to turn even my best friend's alabaster white but to extrapolate that into some sort of hereditary tendency, well it's just a liberty, why St Bernadette herself would turn in her grave. And I know, because I was there as she gasped her dying words "Open my chest and let me breathe!"

But seasons came and went and in 1784, I parted company with Samuel Johnson who was somewhat more profound as he coughed his last words, "It matters not how a man dies, but how he lives. The act of dying is not of importance, it lasts so short a time." And then in October 1820, short of some intellectual conversation, I went to Rome with the English romantic poet, John Keats for a holiday. John was one of the main figures of the second generation of Romantic poets, along with Lord Byron and Percy Bysshe Shelley, despite the fact his works had been in publication for only four years. There were rumours circulating in England that he wanted to leave me at home, but we shared a house at the foot of the Spanish steps until we parted company on February 23rd, 1821 as he died in the arms of his friend Joseph Severn. John was only 25 years of age but already famous.

At this stage, I had got a taste for the Mediterranean vitae in the company of artisans, so in 1838, I left again for my winter holidays to Majorca. This time it was with Frederic Chopin, who was anything but discrete and he went around the island coughing so much that the locals got suspicious and followed him to the old Carthusian monastery of Valdemosa. Few know, it was here that Chopin produced some of his best nocturnes, including the poetically colourful, '24 Preludes op. 28'. But not happy with doing that, he bribed his way out of the monastery and left on a passenger ship to Spain, where he haemoptysised upon his fellow passengers. This young Romanticist who had wrote Polish mazurkas about chasing peasant girls and hunting partridges was immediately put ashore and had to take a pig transporter onwards. The gentile composer of youthful rondos, polonaises and concertos, the man who had heralded the coming harmonies of Wagner, reduced to travel with pigs, just because he kept my company. And when the poor man eventually reached Paris, fresh with the latest Paco Porcine, it's little wonder his final words were, "The earth is suffocating, swear to make them cut me open, so I won't be buried alive." Anyway, I'll tell you a story about the windswept Yorkshire moors, for it was there lived the Bronte sisters. And as the winds blew and the gales howled, the family closed their doors to the outside world and just delicately coughed over each other. Then as Maria, Elizabeth and Patrick died in turn, they decided they might as well keep their silence.

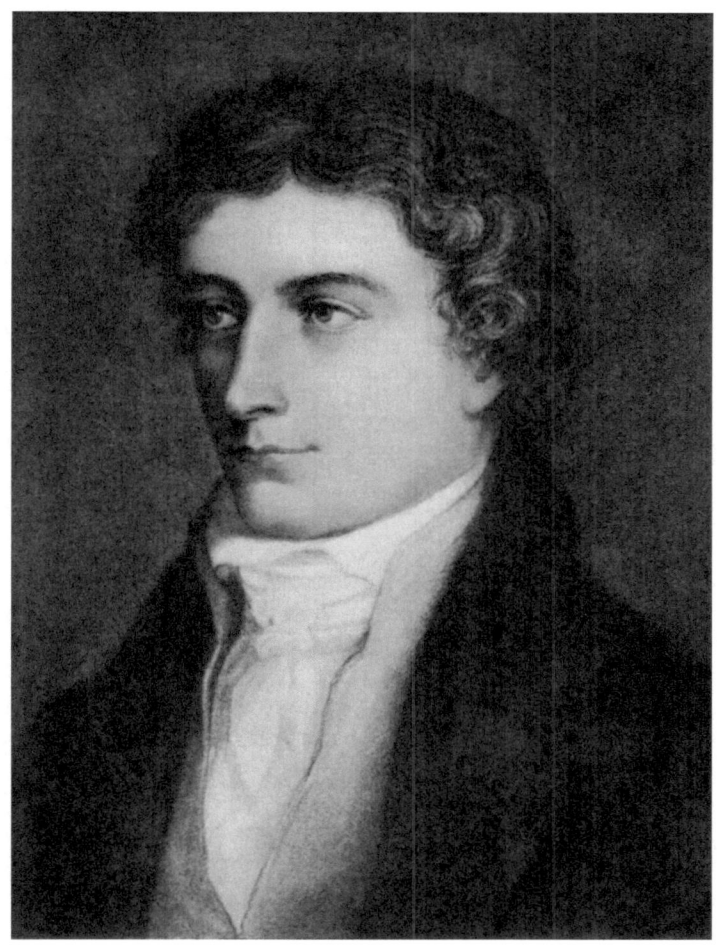

John Keats, (1795–1821), English Poet, Portrait, Illustration

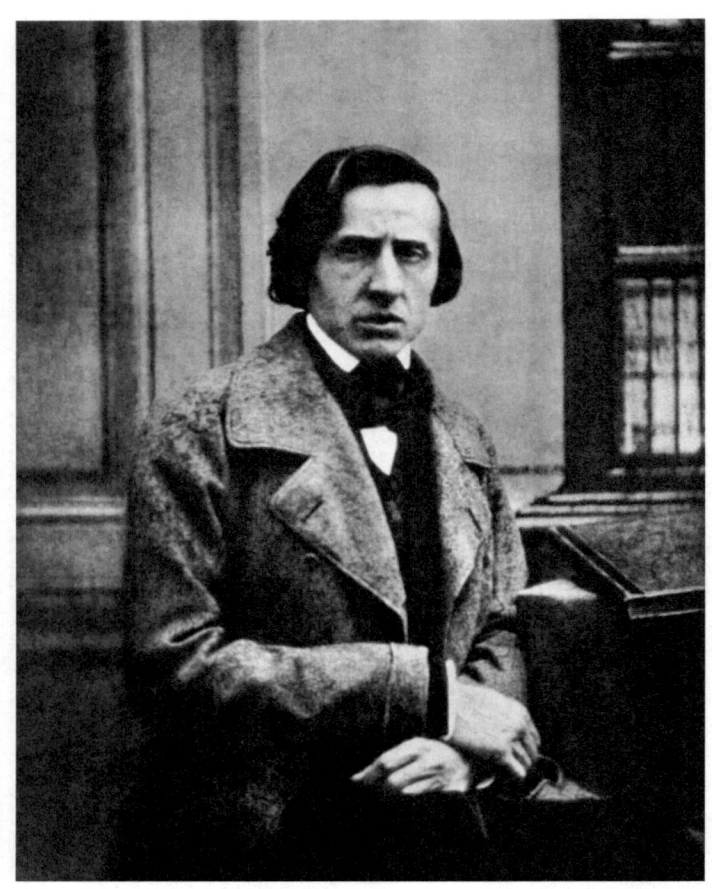

Portrait of the Polish composer and pianist, Frédéric François Chopin (1810–1849), by Louis-Auguste Bisson, c.1849.

When Anne finally died, her parting sentence was meant to strengthen her one surviving sibling "Take courage, Charlotte, take courage!"

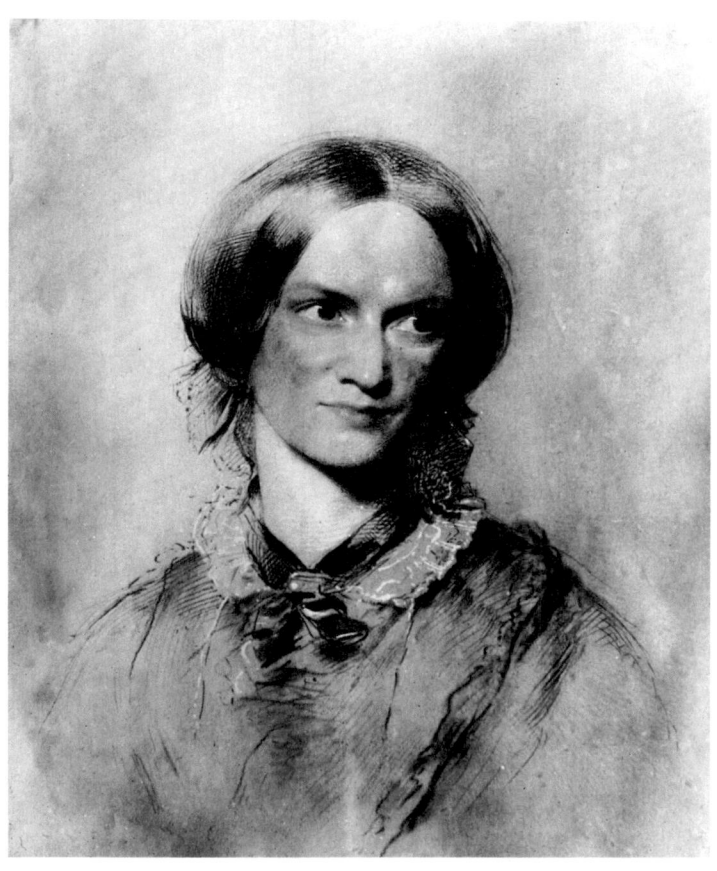

Charlotte Bronte (1816–55) English novelist. Author of 'Jane Eyre' (1847), 'Shirley' (1849), 'Vilette' (1852) Portrait by George Richmond (1809–1896) English artist.

Charlotte, the most prolific writer of the family, got married before she died, and her death certificate was recorded as 'phthisis' the Greek word for the consumption. In fact, Hippocrates used the term, but as he is in the doghouse for giving the Swedes a bad name, I will not extrapolate. Then in 1882, Robert Koch, a country doctor from the Rhineland, tried to convince everybody that the wriggling red microbes that he observed under his microscope were the cause of consumption and that I was readily identifiable with a crimson stain. His giggling colleagues put his theories of socialist bugs to rest and one year later, Sir Walter Scott fell for my charms. Four years later, Doc Holliday went to Glenwood Springs to see if the sulphur vapours would improve his cough, but he was too far gone and on November 8, 1887, he asked for a glass of whiskey. Then he said, "This is funny," and died. He always believed that his end would come from lead poisoning, at the end of a rope, but lost his biggest bet when he died of tuberculosis.

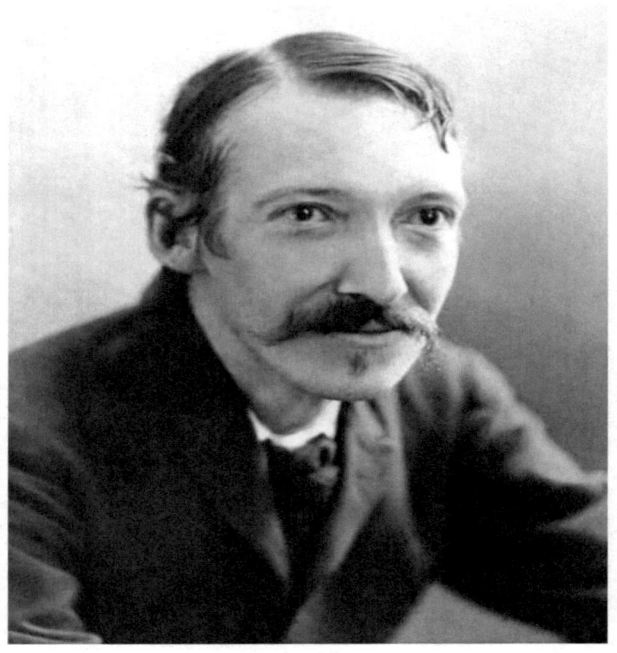

Robert Louis Stevenson (1850–1894) Scottish travel writer and novelist in 1893. Photo: Henry Barnett

As the decade passed, I befriended Robert Louis Stevenson, while he mixed in London literary circles, receiving encouragement from W. E. Henley, whom may have provided the model for Long John Silver in Treasure Island. In 1890, he settled in Samoa where his writing turned away from romance and adventure toward a darker realism. We eventually went our separate ways near Apia, in the Solomon Isles in early December 1894.

In 1888, Selman Abraham Waksman was born in Priluka, near Kiev, Russia, the same year that Rimsky-Korsakov released his colourful composition, Scheherazade. Well, the new century came, and I watched the burial of Cecil John Rhodes. By 1902, he had coughed his last and his final train journey through

Africa to the Matopos Hills was a triumphal affair. Meanwhile, Anton Chekov started coughing up blood and died a few years later.

In 1911, Waksman received a BSc degree in agriculture from Rutgers College and was appointed research assistant in soil bacteriology at the New Jersey Agricultural Experiment Station, where he mostly studied microbes of the soil. As the Great War broke out, D. H. Lawrence escaped conscription because of his chest.

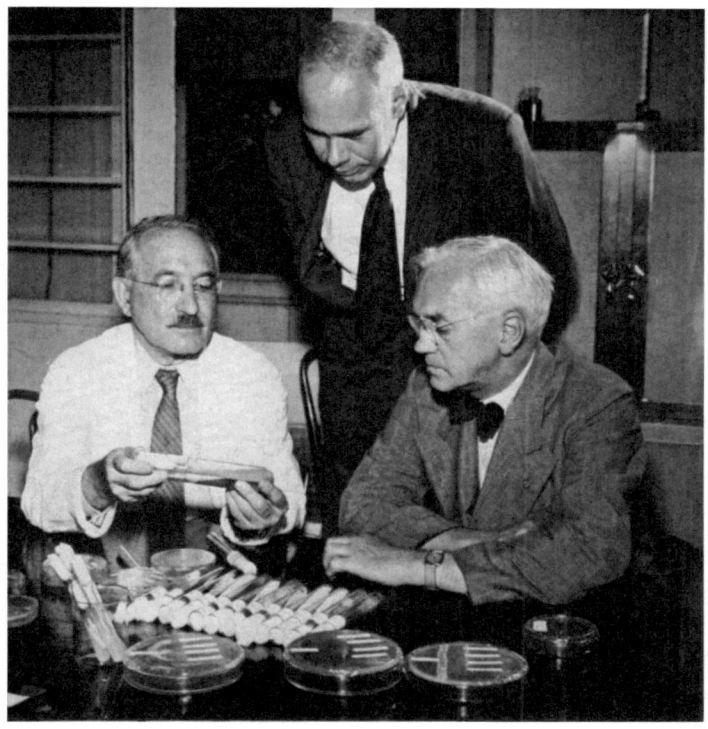

Selman Waksman (left) talking to Sir Alexander Fleming (right) and Randolph T. Major (standing). Fleming (1881–1955) won the Nobel Prize in Physiology or Medicine in 1945 for the discovery of penicillin. Waksman (1888–1973) won the same prize in 1952 for the discovery of streptomycin.

In 1916, Waksman was appointed a research fellow at the University of California where he received his PhD in biochemistry two years later. In 1924, Prague born writer, Franz Kafka, lay haemorrhaging from his lungs in a downtown Vienna hospital. He begged for the doctors to give him a lethal dose of morphine, and in true Wildean fashion screamed to them, "Kill me, or else you are a murderer." In that same year, over 200,000 Americans died of the disease, which was more than the total for heart disease and cancer combined.

Waksman returned to Rutgers as was appointed professor in 1930. It was the same year, an impoverished D.H. Lawrence coughed his last breath in Venice. Over the next few years, he began testing the actinomycetes group for antibiotic activity. He and his co-workers tested about 10,000 microbes for antibiotic activity. In 1940, they isolated actinomycin (1940), the same year Florey managed to isolate and produce a large enough quantity of penicillin to test it on patients. In 1942, they isolated both clavacin, streptothricin, but the great majority of these were unsuitable for medical use, either being too poisonous or failing to meet the special requirements needed for a pharmaceutical drug. Researchers in this period began to feel rather despondent, and many felt that penicillin was unique in the field of antibiotics.

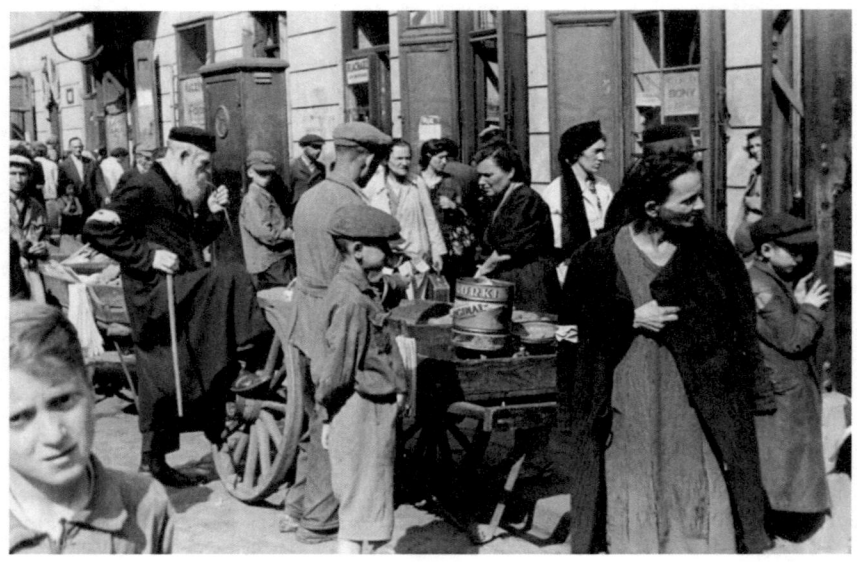

The Warsaw Ghetto was infested with tuberculosis. Dated 1945

During these years I found many friends in Europe and in 1943 it was estimated that I had befriended 100.000 people in the Warsaw ghettos. A similar number were infected in Americans and by the Christmas of that year about half that number had paid the ultimate price. But the tide of life, brought new advances and things were slowly beginning to turn against me. In that same year, Waksman isolated a bacterium called actinomyces griseus in some soil from the

Andes in South America. This bacterium produced a substance that killed many of the bacteria unaffected by penicillin, including the tubercle bacillus. He named the product, *streptomycin*, after the microbe streptomyces griseus, in which it was found. It was part of a chemical group called aminoglycosides, which weakened or killed bacteria by interfering with the process by which they made proteins. The discovery of a substance effective against the tubercle bacillus was a great morale booster to doctors, who were beginning to think there might be some peculiar feature of this bacterium that rendered it immune to chemotherapy. It was not long before they were disappointed when it was discovered that after an interval the tubercle bacilli became resistant to the new drug. Research showed that another drug, sulfetrone, appeared to prevent, or at least delay, the development of this resistance.

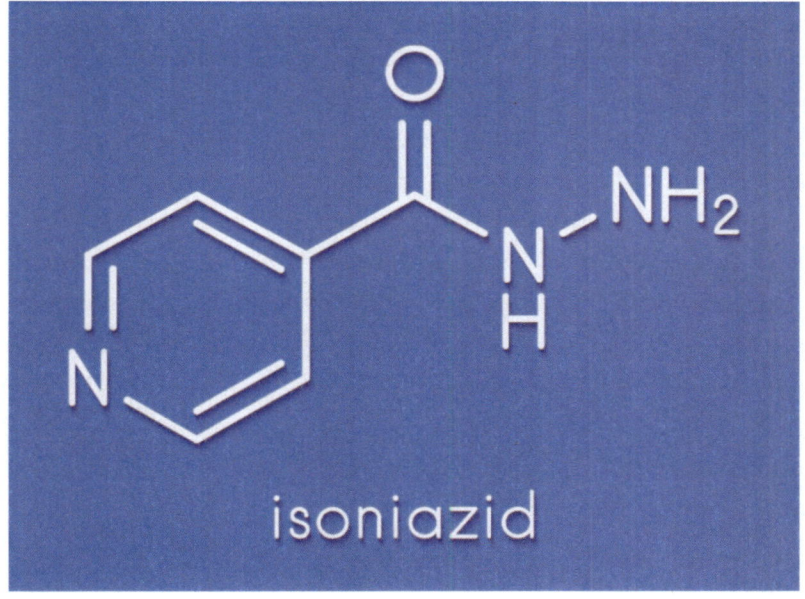

In 1951, isoniazid was added to the anti-tuberculosis pharmacy

November 1944 saw the introduction of streptomycin and an eventual decrease in the number of people that I bestowed friendship on. Waksman's team continued their work and isolated grisein (1946), neomycin (1948), and later fradicin and candicidin, which all had limited effect. A French drug called paraaminosalicylic acid (PAS), appeared to be more effective at preventing resistance and replaced sulfetrone. In 1949, as the victorious Russians were turning the eastern part of Germany into a communist state, Waksman was appointed director of the Institute of microbiology.

In 1951, isoniazid was added to the anti-tuberculosis pharmacy. The substance had been known for some time but was first cautiously used by doctors at the Seaview Hospital in New York. But the treatment of tuberculosis still failed to produce the rapid cure seen in other diseases. This was because the bacilli formed tubercles of dead tissue, which were not easily penetrated and thus the bacilli were protected. In 1952, Waksman was given the Nobel Prize for Medicine, for the discovery of streptomycin and retired six years later at the age of 70 years.

Streptomycin will always be remembered as the first antibiotic effective against tuberculosis, a disease, which once ranked among the most common causes of death in the world. Waksman died in 1973, leaving only one son, Byron, who was then a professor of microbiology at Yale University Medical School. Today, thanks to his efforts, improved treatment has greatly reduced both the number of people who get the disease and the number of people who die from it. However, tuberculosis remains a major concern in developing countries where these improved methods of therapy are not widely available or not properly complied with. There was some controversy about the 1952 Nobel prize in medicine, awarded solely to Selman Waksman for his discovery of streptomycin, omitted the recognition some felt due to his co-discoverer Albert Schatz. This resulted in litigation brought by Schatz against Waksman over the credit of the streptomycin discovery; Schatz was awarded a substantial settlement, and, together with Waksman, Schatz was to be officially recognized as a co-discoverer of streptomycin as concerned patent rights, but he is still not a Nobel Prize laureate.

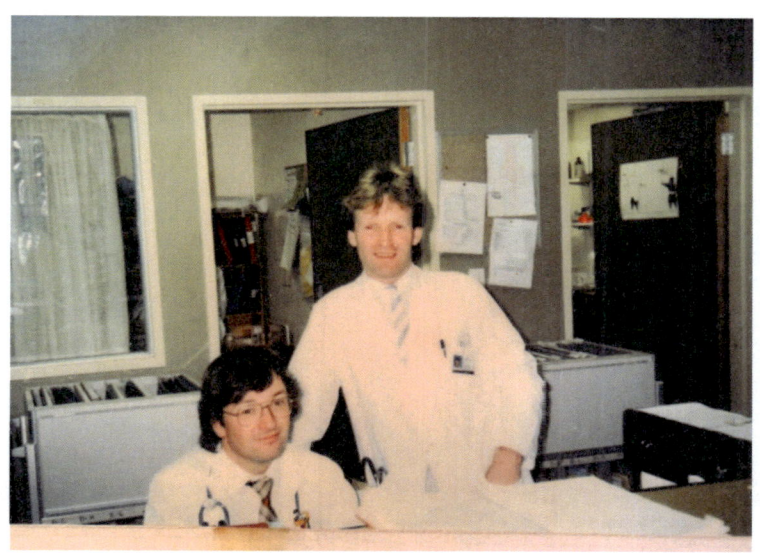

Working with Vietnamese boat people with tuberculosis patients in Dunedin Public Hospital New Zealand

New Zealand is aiming to be the first country in the world to eliminate tuberculosis and have proposed TB elimination strategy based on the eight-point World Health Organization (WHO) action framework for low incidence countries. However, it was different when I worked there in 1987. In 1975, the South Vietnamese capital Saigon fell to the Viet Cong and the North Vietnamese forces after decades of war in Vietnam, in 1975. This brought great social upheaval with a mass exodus of Vietnamese people fearing what life would be like under a new Communist government. During the late 1970s and early 1980s, many Vietnamese risked everything to escape. These refugees were called 'boat people' because they fled their war-ravaged country in crowded boats and carried all their diseases, including viral hepatitis B, leprosy, and tuberculosis with them. During these perilous journeys, they suffered ill health, food shortages, piracy, rape, and murder. On arrival in New Zealand, they were placed in camps to await official refugee status, which allowed them to apply for permanent resettlement and have their diseases treated. Greenlane Hospital in Auckland and Dunedin Public Hospital were chosen as the relevant tuberculosis centres for each island.

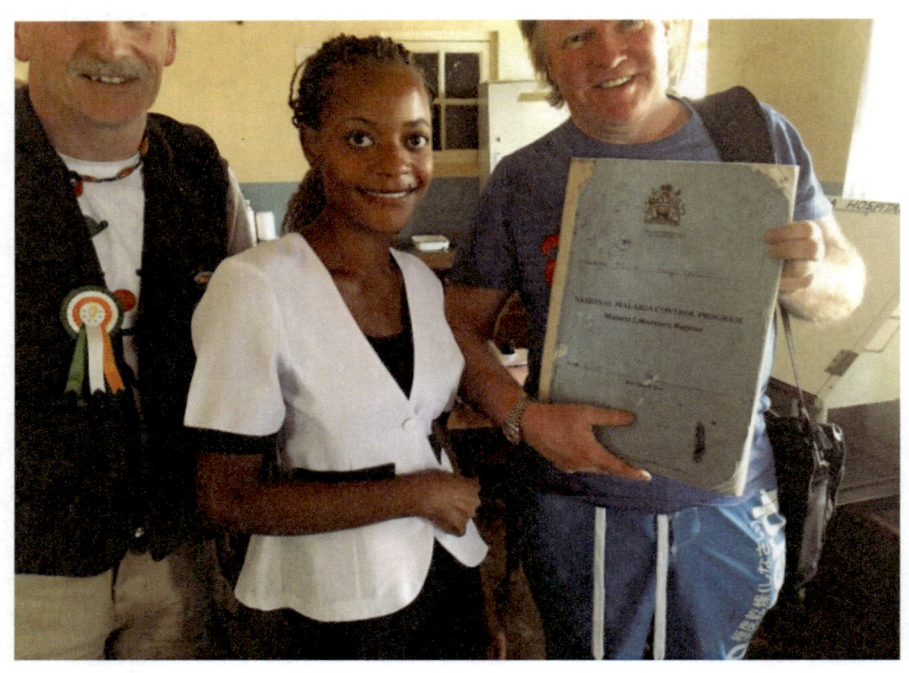

The author with fellow humanitarian Peter Gannon and nurse checking out the old TB Register in Mau Hospital, Malawi in 2016

I Am *Plasmodium Vivax*, Destroyer of the Roman Empire

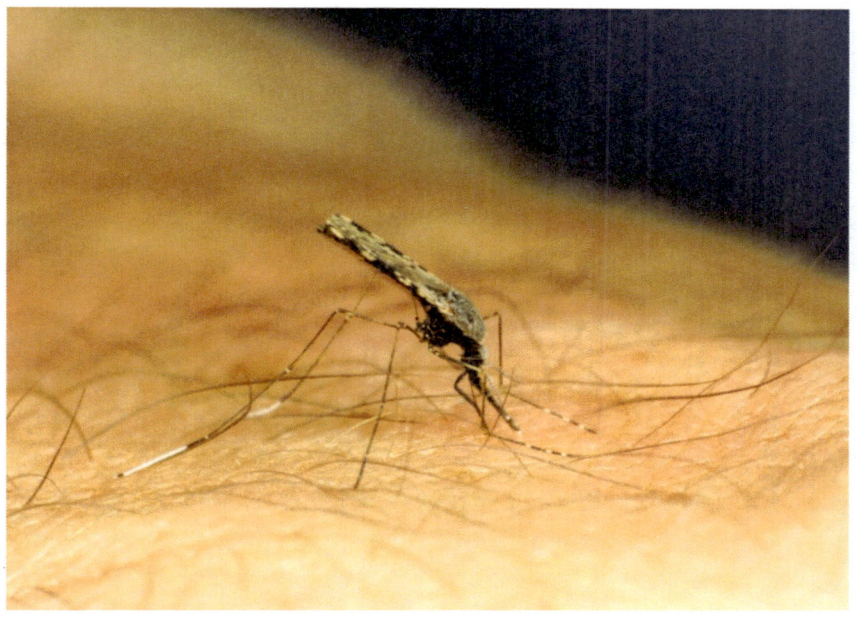

Plasmodium vivax is a protozoal parasite and a human pathogen. This parasite is the most frequent and widely distributed cause of recurring malaria. It is primarily transmitted through the bite of infected Anopheles mosquitoes. P. vivax is one of the five species of Plasmodium that can infect humans and is responsible for a significant portion of malaria cases worldwide. Although it is less virulent than Plasmodium falciparum, the deadliest of the five human malaria parasites, P. vivax malaria infections can lead to severe disease and death, often due to splenomegaly. P. vivax is carried by the female Anopheles mosquito; the males do not bite. Malaria caused by P. vivax is characterized by recurrent fever episodes, which can occur at 48-hour intervals. Other common symptoms

include chills, headache, fatigue, and muscle aches. Unlike some other malaria species, P. vivax can form dormant liver stages called hypnozoites, which can cause relapses months or even years after the initial infection. The global distribution of P. vivax malaria is widespread, particularly in regions of Asia, Latin America, and the Western Pacific. It poses a significant public health burden and can contribute to anemia, organ damage, and complications during pregnancy.

Treatment for P. vivax malaria typically involves a combination of antimalarial medications. In addition to treatment, preventive measures such as insecticide-treated bed nets, indoor residual spraying, and chemoprophylaxis are important in controlling the spread of the disease.

This is my story.

I am Plasmodium vivax, a small protozoan carried about by Anopheles airlines to every man in every humid city that sleeps in the sunset. In fact, our transportation system is so effective that once nearly three-quarters of the known world was serviced by our pilots, which was surprising seeing that only pregnant females could apply for the position. Well, political correctness aside, I've led an interesting life to date. If you read the Iliad again, you will realise that it was me who struck down the Greek forces at the siege of Troy. And it was the Greek soldiers that carried me across Asia, why they say I was even directly involved in the death of Alexander the Great. But it was not just the Greeks who battled the constant problems of chronic malaria and let a Golden Age disappear from their midst because fewer people know I was involved in the fall of The Roman Empire. In the 1st Century BC, during the years of Julius Caesar's campaigns, over sixty percent of the population of Rome was incapacitated with chronic illness that I had spread in their midst. The great Caesar himself and many of his soldiers fell to the ravages that I brought. Columella, in his twelve-volume work on farming and agriculture theory wrote about how fatigue from chronic malaria greatly curtailed efforts of the farmers to produce enough food for the Roman population, which was growing in the period. At one time, all of Campagna, which produced fresh vegetables for the city had to stop production as I had not left an able-bodied man to continue supplies. The stricken farmers went to Rome for help and carried me along with them. The infant mortality soared, and life expectancy sharply declined. It is written that the bad Roman airs 'malaria' are supposed to have plagued the city for another five hundred years. In 165, Galen himself tried to treat people that I had visited and accordingly recorded his efforts. The epidemic raged for fifteen years and took the life of the Emperor, Marcus Aurelius. Few know by the fourth century most of Roman's soldiers started to be recruited from lands, far in the north, where I found it too cold to live in. It is thought by myself, that my weakening influence, more so than any alleged decadence of the Roman citizens caused the fall of the Great Empire. Refugees came and went, and by the time of the Crusades, malaria had gripped most of the continent. And if that wasn't enough, it followed the new colonialists across the Atlantic, all the way to America. Before long, over half the population of New England suffered from chills, fevers and exhaustion caused by a condition known as the ague. Well, that was just me with a new American accent. By the time of the Revolution, I had spread my wings to such an extent that George Washington grew seriously worried about the condition of his troops. The rumour went around that the bad air in the cities was causing the illness and millions decided to throw caution to the wind and head for the plains of the mid-west. But they should have known better, for in 1822, nine hundred of the thousand citizens of Columbus, Ohio were shaking with the ague. By 1833, ninety-thousand of the one hundred and fifty thousand settlers around the town were infected.

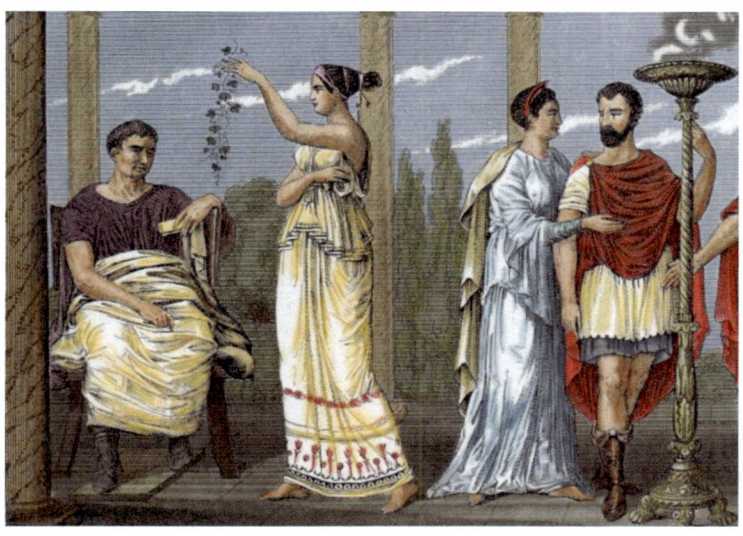

Scene from the Roman Empire at its height of power

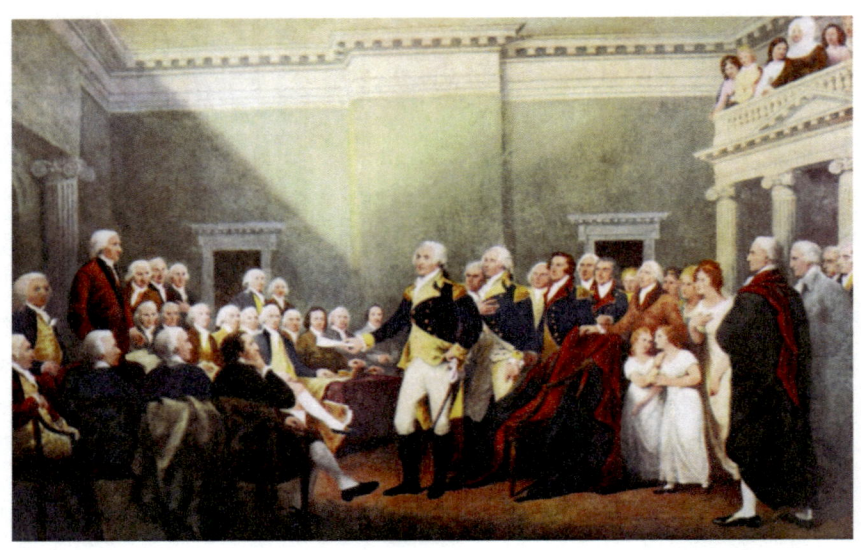

Washington Resigning Command of the Army

In 1857, Ronald Ross was born in Almora, on the Indian subcontinent. It was the same year as the Sepoy revolt that led to the formation of British India. He studied medicine at St Bartholomew's and entered the Indian Medical Service in 1881. One year later, he became interested in the study of malaria, determined to prove the hypothesis of Scottish physician and parasitologist, Sir Patrick Manson who was convinced that mosquitoes were related to the propagation of the disease. Manson was a founder of the field of tropical medicine. He graduated from the University of Aberdeen with degrees in Master of Surgery, Doctor of Medicine and Doctor of Law.

In 1897, Ross finally demonstrated the lifecycle of malarial parasites in mosquitoes, and two years later he returned to England and joined the Liverpool School of Tropical Medicine under the direction of Sir Alfred Jones. He was immediately sent to West Africa to continue his investigations into the species of mosquitoes that convey African fever.

In 1901, he was elected a fellow of the Royal College of Surgeons of England and a fellow of the Royal Society, of which he was vice president from 1911 to 1913. In 1902, he was appointed professor of tropical medicine in Liverpool, and physician for tropical diseases at Kings College Hospital, London, 10 years later.

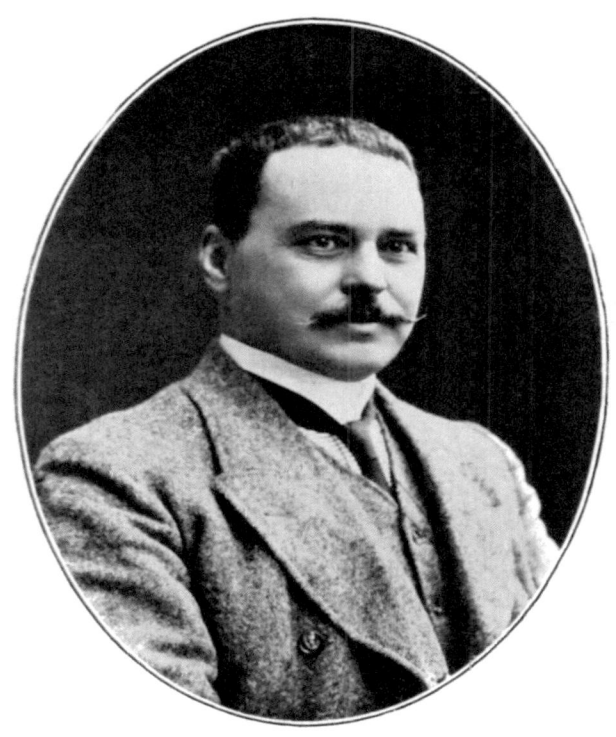

Sir Ronald Ross, a British medical doctor who received the Nobel Prize for Physiology or Medicine in 1902 for his work on the transmission of malaria.

He presented a report on malaria in Mauritius in 1908, and his work, *Prevention of Malaria*, three years later. These were elaborated into a more scientific form and published by the Royal Society in 1915 and 1916. These papers represented a profound interest, not confined to epidemiology, but also to pure and applied mathematics. He remained in his tropical medicine posts until 1917, when he consulted on epidemic malaria in combatant troops, a position which was later recognised by his elevation to the order of St George in 1918.

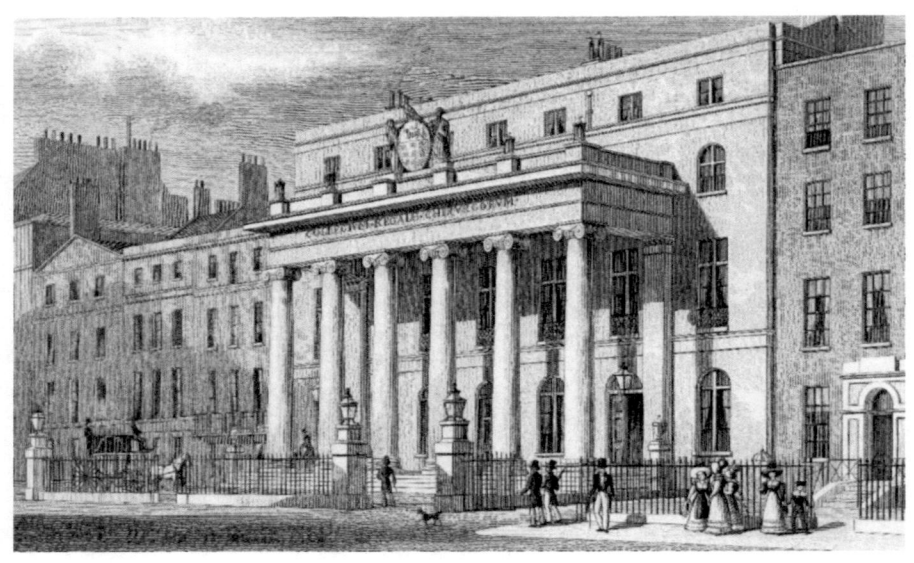

The Royal College of Surgeons of England, London, illustration by Shepherd, 1826

He received an honorary MD degree in Stockholm in 1910, and when his memoirs were published in 1923, he dedicated them to the people of Sweden and the memory of Alfred Nobel. Ross became president of the Society of Tropical Medicine and used his position to try and prevent malaria in different countries of the world. About the turn of the century, a medical officer by the name of Charles Laveran was soaking up the heat of the Algerian sun and noticed me waving at him from under his microscope. For some reason, he suspected that I had been secretly hitching around on Anopheles airways for the past few thousand years. Luckily, his friends were still into the four humours theory of life and it took another seventeen years before British physician, Ronald Ross found me stowing away inside an Anopheline baggage compartment.

Ross initiated schemes in West Africa, the Suez Canal, Greece, Cyprus, and the areas affected by the 1914–1918 war. He also tried to prevent malaria within the planting industries of India and Ceylon. He made many contributions to the epidemiology of malaria, including the development of mathematical models which remain the basis of much of the understanding of insect-borne diseases. Well, a call went out on all the airlines until an Italian zoologist, G.B. Crazzi found out that I only travelled with Anopheles and needed human blood every three days to nourish her young. He also discovered that the mosquito only feeds at night; well, before long my game was up, although it is documented that in the year 1948, I visited over three hundred thousand people of which about three million died. And that's only an average because in some countries such as India as many as thirteen million people were stricken annually, with the total population of Ireland dying each year. There is no doubt about it, my influence has changed the direction of the world.

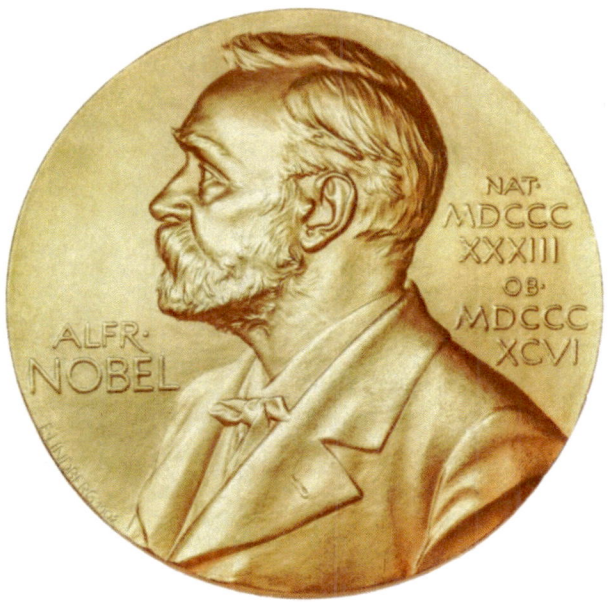

Ross received many honours including the Nobel Prize in 1902 and was given honorary membership of learned societies of most countries. His single-minded search for truth caused friction with many people, but nevertheless he enjoyed a vast circle of friends throughout the world. He also found time for other pursuits, being poet, playwright, writer, and painter. His poetic works gained him wide acclamation which was independent of his medical and mathematical standing. Ronald Ross married Rosa Bessie Bloxam in 1889. They had two sons – Ronald and Charles – and two daughters – Dorothy and Sylvia. His wife died in 1931, and Ross died a year later, the same year that Amelia Earhart made history after landing her Lockheed Vega at Culmore, Northern Ireland.

Malaria is caused by Plasmodium parasites. The parasites are spread to people through the bites of infected female Anopheles mosquitoes, called 'malaria vectors'. There are five parasite species that cause malaria in humans, and two of these species – *P. falciparum* and *P. vivax* – pose the greatest threat. In 2018, *P. falciparum* accounted for 99.7% of estimated malaria cases in the WHO African Region. *P. vivax* is the predominant parasite in the WHO Region of the Americas, representing 75% of malaria cases. *Anopheles gambiae* is the vector of transmission in Liberia.

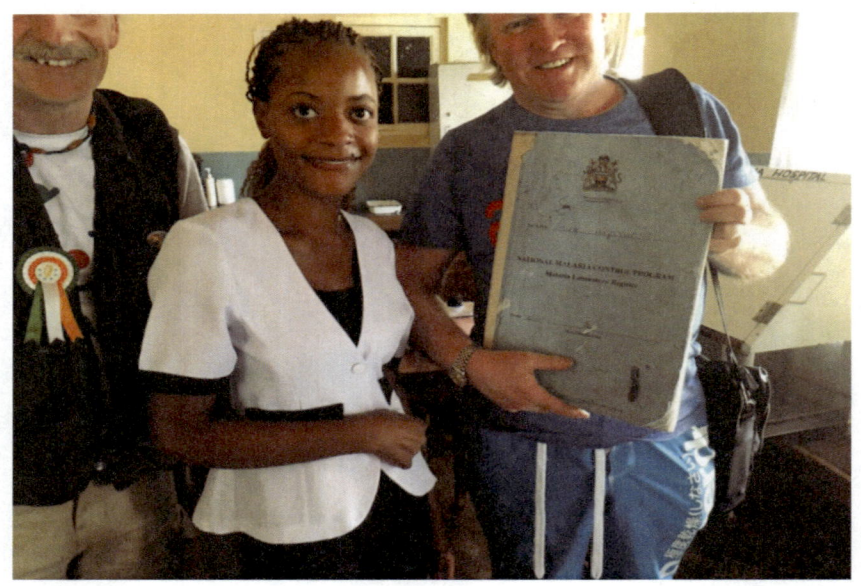

The author at a malaria clinic in Malawi

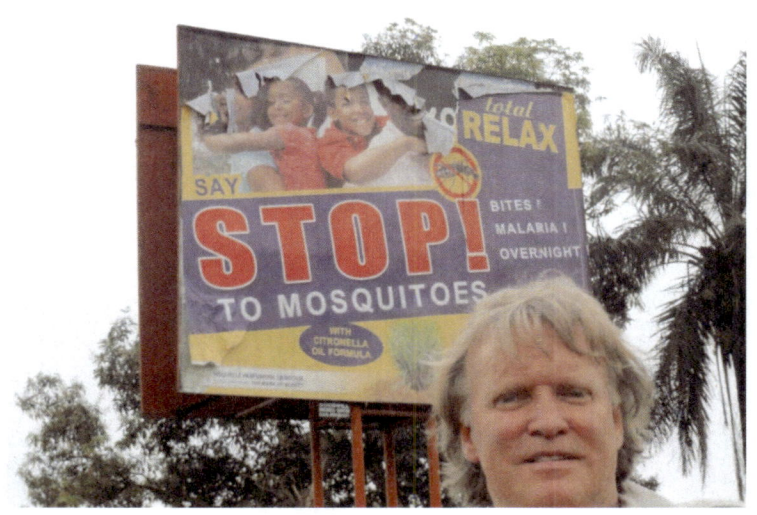

The author on a humanitarian mission in Liberia in 2012

Key Facts

- Malaria is a life-threatening disease caused by parasites that are transmitted to people through the bites of infected female Anopheles mosquitoes. It is preventable and curable.
- In 2019, there were an estimated 229 million cases of malaria worldwide. The estimated number of malaria deaths stood at 409,000.
- Children aged under 5 years are the most vulnerable group affected by malaria, they account for 67% (274,000) of all malaria deaths worldwide.
- The WHO African Region carries a disproportionately high share of the global malaria burden. In 2019, the region was home to 94% of malaria cases and deaths.

I Am *Vibrio Cholerae*, and I Changed the World by Improving Sanitation

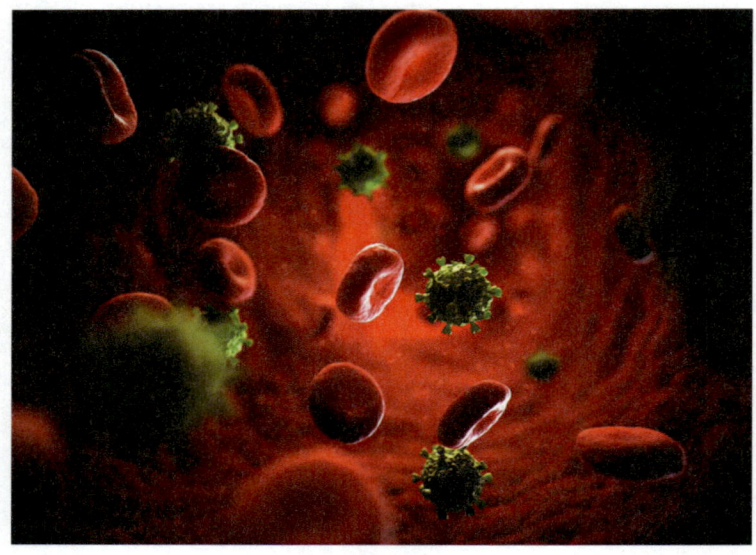

Vibrio cholerae is a Gram-negative, comma-shaped bacterium. The bacterium's natural habitat is brackish or saltwater where they attach themselves easily to the chitin-containing shells of crabs, shrimps, and other shellfish.

I am Vibrio cholerae and have been around since first being described in the ancient Sanskrit text, the *Sushruta Samhita* over two thousand years ago. While this important text of Satapatha Brahmana has some status due to its chapters describing surgical training, I was even more impressed to get an honourable mention by the 'Father of Medicine', Greek physician Hippocrates, who was given this title as he was the first westerner to separate medicine from the other intellectual pursuits of philosophy and theology. As well as being credited with coining the Hippocratic Oath, which is still relevant and used in medicine today, he described me in detail, observing a gastrointestinal disease process associated with drinking contaminated water. There is little doubt, I started my journey in life in India, most probably around the banks of the Ganges Delta. In fact, Kolkata city, the capital city of West Bengal state in the delta has been described as the 'homeland of cholera'. And don't for a moment think of only inhabiting slums and areas of hunger, as this city is allegedly home to 10, 000 millionaires and 5 billionaires with a total wealth of nearly $0.3 trillion.

I am mentioned by the Portuguese historian, Gaspar Correia who wrote a book in 1543 about Asiatic cholera, mentioning that during infection, I cause profuse, watery diarrhoea. It would be many more years before they would discover this was caused by my endotoxin. While mentioning Gaspar, he ended up being murdered by order of Governor Estevao da Gama, who was the son of Vasco da Gama, the Portuguese explorer who discovered the sea route to India, via the Cape of Good Hope. The Portuguese discovery of vital importance as it was the first recorded trip directly from Europe to India and enabled the Portuguese to become the leading country in Europe for almost one hundred years and establish a colonial empire in Kerala and around the Indian Ocean.

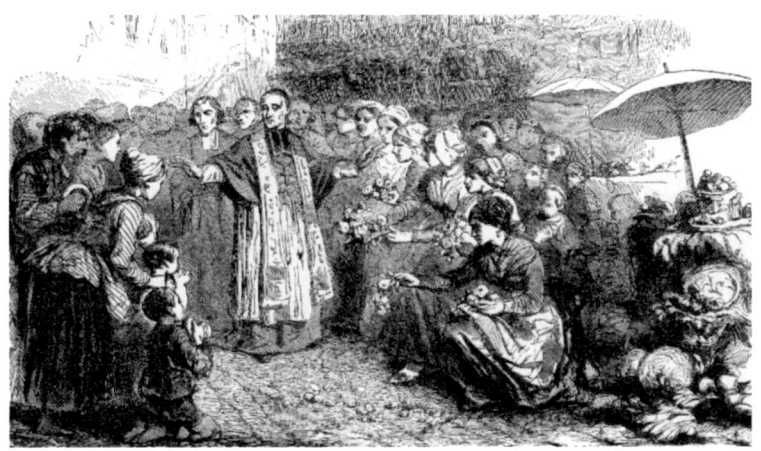

A procession of Pope Gregory XVI, 1765–1846, during the cholera epidemic in Italy

My first major claim to fame occurred in 1817, when I appeared in Jessore, a city in the Jashore District, located in the south-western region of Bangladesh. Incidentally, it was the same year that the New York Stock Exchange opened. I quickly spread through most of the neighbouring countries, and by 1820, I was in Thailand, Indonesia, and the Philippines. It is estimated that I was responsible for the deaths of 100,000 people on the island of Java alone.

I made my way to China in 1820 and Japan in 1822 by way of infected people on ships.

The pandemic died out in 1823, possibly thanks to a severe winter in 1823–1824, which may have killed the bacteria living in the frozen water supplies. By autumn of 1830, cholera I made it to Moscow, and then in spring of 1831, reached Finland and Poland. It then passed into Hungary and Germany. I decided to reach England by the winter of 1831 way of returning soldiers passing through the port of Sunderland from India. It appears their ships passed through Oman and the Persian Gulf and spread cholera to Syria and Turkey. Within a few months, I was in London causing uproar and a desire for social change. Nobody knew what caused the illness and most blamed the bad air in the cities. The English public started to distrust scientists and doctors, and just like the present Covid pandemic press misreporting led people to believe patients were being killed in the hospitals to use their bodies for anatomical dissection, an outcome they referred to as 'Burking'. The riots, which began in Russia were caused by the anti-cholera measures, undertaken by the tsarist government, such as quarantine, armed cordons, and travel restrictions.

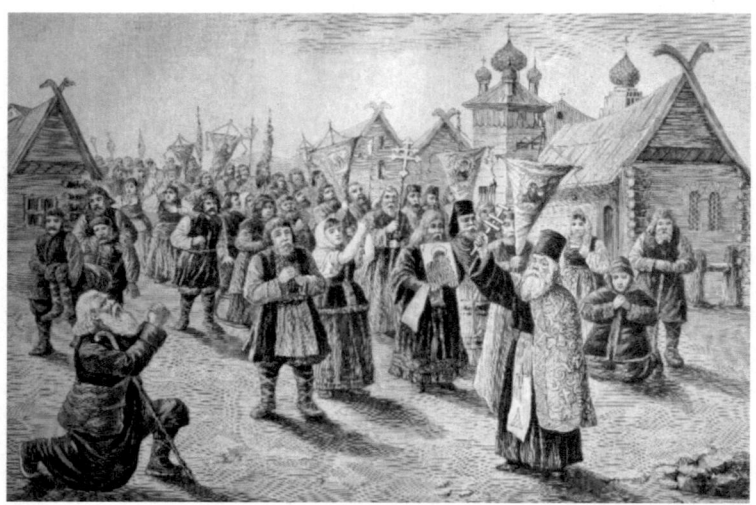

Cholera procession in Russia, historical illustration, ca. 1893

A major riot took place in Aberdeen on 26 December 1831, when a dog dug up a dead body in the city. It is estimated that 20,000 Aberdonians protested against the medical establishment, who they believed were using the epidemic as a body-snatching scheme similar to the Burke and Hare murders of 1828. On August 29, 1909, The New York Times reported more cholera riots in Russia. The city of Liverpool experienced more riots than elsewhere. In 1832, major street riots occurred against the local medical doctors, the protestors convinced that cholera victims were being removed to the hospital to be killed by doctors in order to use them for anatomical dissection. 'Bring out the Barkers' was one cry of the Liverpool mobs, referring to the Burke and Hare scandal four years earlier, when two men had murdered people in Edinburgh in order to sell their bodies for dissection to the local anatomy school.

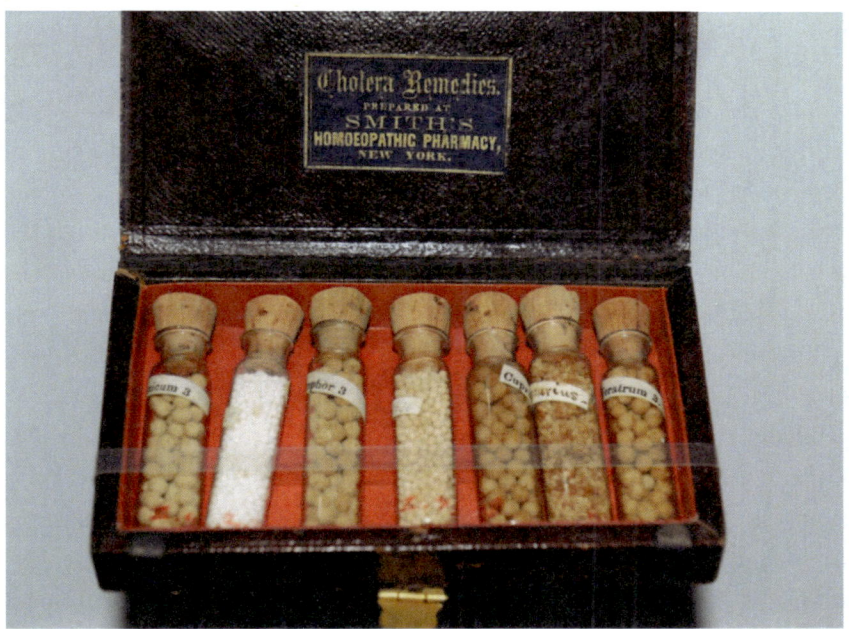

Box of homeopathic remedies, 1870–1900, for treating cholera

In 1832, cholera had also made it to the Americas. Beginning my journey with Quebec, saw 1,000 deaths from the disease, I quickly spread along the St Lawrence River and its tributaries, killing thousands of people. Then, I made my way through New York and Miami to reach Latin America, including Mexico and Cuba by 1833. It was the same year that The United Kingdom claimed sovereignty over the Falkland Islands and The Slavery Abolition Act received Royal Assent, abolishing slavery through most the British Empire. More cholera pandemics occurred in the periods 1863–1875 and 1881–1896, but they were less severe than previous outbreaks. Between 1872 and 1873, Hungary suffered 190,000 deaths from cholera. In 1854, as I claimed 23,000 people in Great Britain, the bacterium Vibrio cholerae was first isolated as the cause of the illness by Italian microbiologist Filippo Pacini. He correctly identified the cholera bacterium—naming it *cholerigenic vibrios*, and this was done independently at the same time by the Catalan Joaquim Balcells I Pascual.

In 1883, German microbiologist Robert Koch, the founder of modern bacteriology, studied cholera in Egypt and Calcutta, and he developed a technique that allowed him to grow and describe *V. cholerae*. He was able to show that the presence of the bacterium in intestines causes cholera and he publicised both the knowledge and the means of fighting the disease.

In the same year, a British physician and hygienist called John Snow tried to stop me from spreading any further, when he realised that I was squatting in a particular water pump in London's Soho neighbourhood. It is said he would only drink distilled water as he trusted it to be pure. John also had an interest in anaesthesia, and a few years earlier had published a short work entitled '*On the inhalation of the vapour of ether*'. Before the discovery of *Vibrio cholerae*, Snow realised that chloroform was much more potent than ether and required precision when administering it. After a 15-year-old patient, Hannah Greener, died on 28 January 1848 after getting a simple surgical procedure to cut her toenail, he realized that chloroform had to be administered carefully and published his findings in a letter to The Lancet. In continuing his pursuit of medical hygiene and interest in cholera, he focused on that pump in London. To be fair to him, it was a good deduction as nobody realised that I was causing the disease. He used a dot map to illustrate the cluster of cholera cases around my home in the pump and showed that homes supplied by the Southwark and Vauxhall Waterworks Company, had a cholera rate fourteen times that of those supplied by Lambeth Waterworks Company, which obtained cleaner water upriver.

In a letter to the editor of the *Medical Times and Gazette* in 1854, John Snow wrote, "I had an interview with the Board of Guardians of St James's parish and represented the above circumstances to them. In consequence of what I said, the handle of the pump was removed on the following day. A plaque commemorates Snow and his 1854 study in the place of the water pump on Broad Street (now

Broadwick Street). It shows a water pump with its handle removed. The spot where the pump stood is covered with red granite. The sixth cholera pandemic (1899–1923) had less of an effect on Western Europe and North America due to advances in public health and sanitation. But the disease still ravaged India, Russia, the Middle East, and northern Africa. As cholera is caused by ingesting food or water contaminated with a certain bacterium, it overwhelmingly harms countries hampered by extreme wealth inequality and lack of social development. Cholera unfairly hurts the parts of our planet least able to defend themselves, while richer countries barely worry about it anymore. By 1923, cholera cases had dissipated throughout much of the world, except India—it killed more than half a million people in India in both 1918 and 1919. In 1990, more than 90 percent of all cholera cases reported to WHO were from the African continent. In 1991, I came back to Peru, where I had been absent for a hundred years. I killed 3,000 people in Peru and then spread to South and Central America and Mexico. More recently, I visited Zimbabwe affecting 97,000 people and killing 4,200. On October 20, 2010, an outbreak of cholera was confirmed in Haiti for the first time in more than a century, ten months after the catastrophic earthquake that killed over 200,000 people and displaced over 1 million. This cholera outbreak is the worst in recent history with over 665,000 cases and 8,183 deaths. The cholera outbreak spread throughout the country and became endemic, being the first modern large-scale outbreak of cholera. Early efforts were made to cover up the source of the epidemic, but largely due, to the investigations of journalist Jonathan M. Katz and epidemiologist Renaud Piarroux, it is was shown to be the result of contamination by infected United Nations peacekeepers deployed from Nepal."

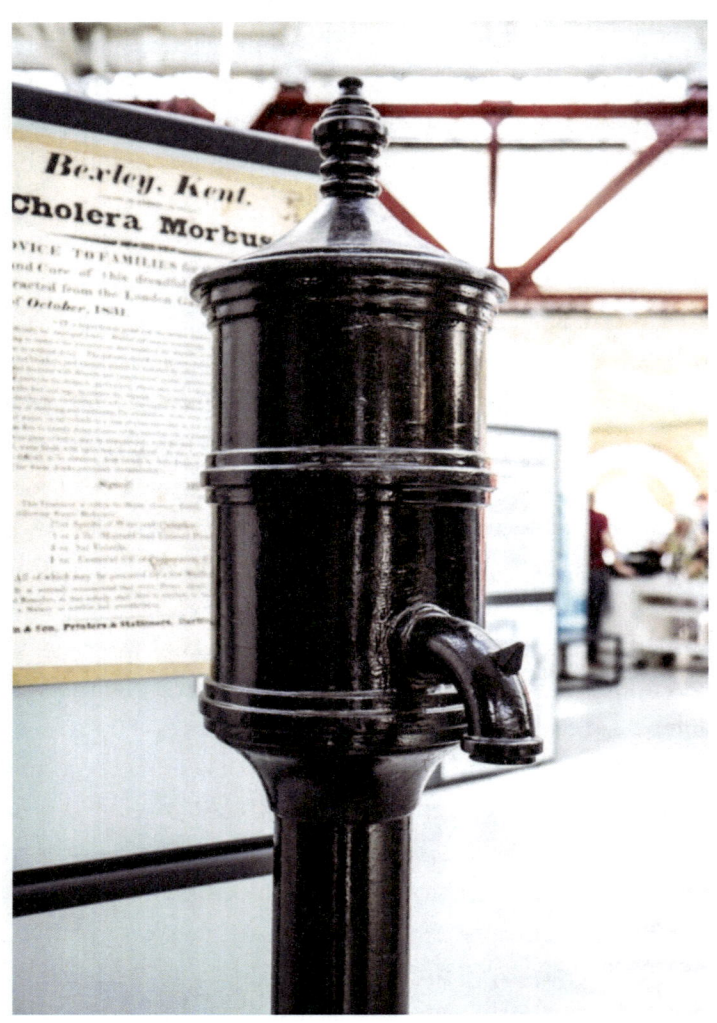

John Snow cholera outbreak water pump on display at the Crossness Pumping Station London sewage system museum, UK

****

In 2017, outbreaks of cholera broke out in Somalia and Yemen. By August 2017, the Yemen outbreak affected 500,000 people and killed 2,000 people. The World Health Organization calls cholera 'the forgotten pandemic' and that it continues to this day. Cholera reportedly affects 1.3 million to 4 million people every year, with annual fatalities ranging from 21,000 to 143,000.

I Am *Treponema pallidum*, Who Sailed with The Slave Ships to America to Cause Syphilis

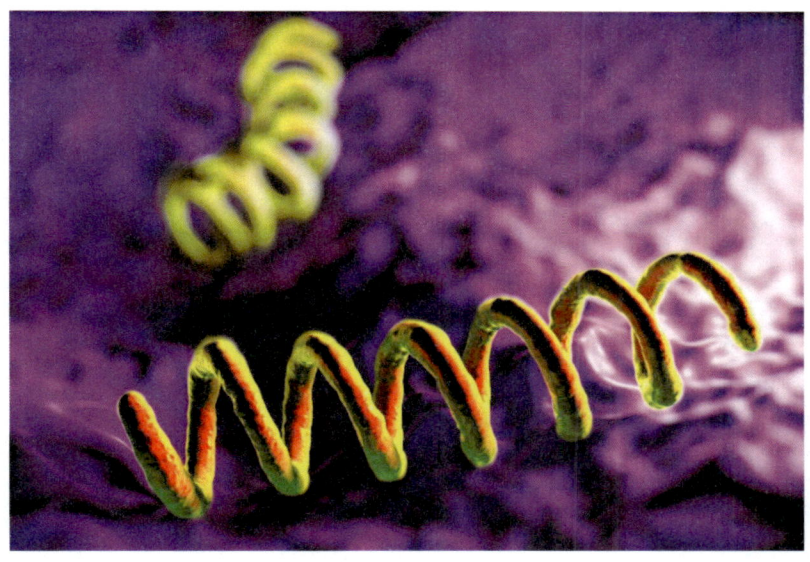

Treponema pallidum **bacteria, computer illustration**

Syphilis is a sexually transmitted disease caused by Treponema Pallidum, a bacterium from the *Spirochaetaceae* family. There are at least three human treponemal diseases causing yaws, pinta and bejel Examination of skeletons show bone alterations distinctive to these diseases, separating them from syphilis, even though current DNA and immunologic technologies find it difficult to recognise the difference. The signs and symptoms of syphilis vary depending on which of the four stages it presents (primary, secondary, latent, and tertiary). The treponemal disease appears to have started in East Africa and spread to England, with the slave trade. The original treponemal disease apparently spread from Africa through Asia, entering North America. Many scientists feel that syphilis and non-venereal treponemal diseases are really variants of the same infections and the clinical differences happen only because of geographic and climate variations, however we do know that *treponema pertenue* causes yaws, *treponema carateum* causes pinta and *treponema pallidum* bejel. These three diseases are not typically sexually transmitted. Either way, within the past eight thousand years later, *treponema* mutated to syphilis.

The term 'syphilis' was introduced by Girolamo Fracastoro, a poet and medical personality in Verona, who wrote a book where Apollo, one of the Olympian deities in classical Greek and Roman religion gets offended and curses people with a hideous disease named syphilis, after the shepherd's name.

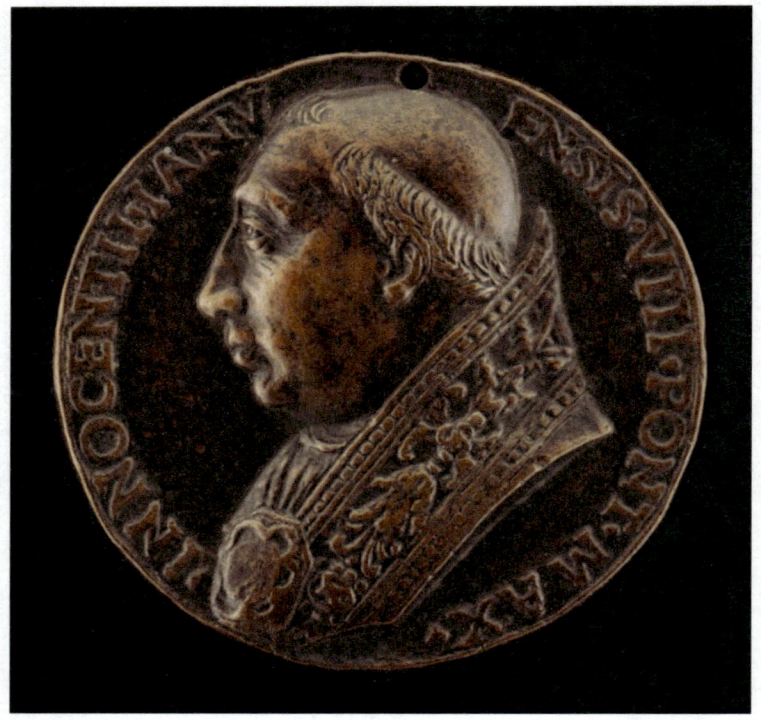

Pope Innocent VIII

I am first mentioned in Europe in the late 15th century and there is good reason to suggest my appearance coincided with the return of Columbus's fleet from the New World. While not giving away any secrets of my past journeys, there is apparent skeletal evidence of myself at the site in the Dominican Republic where Columbus landed. Hence, many say this evidence is consistent with this site as the point of initial contact of syphilis and of its subsequent spread from the New World to the Old. Others say that I was already present in Europe but mistaken for leprosy. These suggestions are called the Columbian and pre-Columbian hypotheses, respectively, with the Columbian hypothesis better supported by better historical and clinical evidence. Either way, Christopher Columbus returned from America in 1493, and within a short period witnessed a French Army invasion of some of the states of Italy. The trouble started a few years before, when Pope Innocent VIII offered the kingdom of Naples to French king Charles VIII, because the Italian king, Ferdinand I refused to pay his debts to him. In 1494, Charles VIII entered Italy with an army of 25,000 men, and wreaked havoc on Rome and Naples, stealing everything they could lay their hands on. The soldiers carried me with them, and I was described by Italian physicians as being worse than leprosy. Not knowing whether to be impressed or not, I was certainly not as fatal as the bubonic plague, though my symptoms were painful and resulted in the appearance of genital sores, and foul abscesses and ulcers over the rest of the body. The remedies to treat me in those days were few and mostly consisted of heavy metals—first mercurial and later arsenic and bismuth preparations, resulting in many patients dying of mercury poisoning. My appearance later proved to be syphilis, and soon I had spread throughout most of Italy.

Documents belonging to Fernandez de Oviedo and Ruy Diaz de Isla, two physicians with Spanish origins state Columbus's sailors brought me from the New World in 1493. Diaz de Isla goes further and writes that an 'unknown disease, so far not seen and never described', appeared in Barcelona in 1493 and originated in Española, part of the Galápagos Islands. He mentions that Pinzon de Palos, the pilot of Columbus, and other crew members suffered from syphilis on their return from the New World. German scholar and poet Ulrich von Hutten wrote in his book, "In the yere of Chryst 1493 or there about, this most foule and most grevous disease beganne to sprede amongst the people." It seemed nobody likes me, and even William Shakespeare's obsessive interest in mentioning me in his poems of the sonnets, as well as his clinical knowledge, suggested to many that he himself may have been infected. He called me 'the infinite malady', and recognised I was a disease, worthy of disgrace and great disapproval. It is said that in England, Italy, and Germany, I was called it 'the French disease', while the Russians called me the 'Polish disease', the Turks coined the term 'Christian disease', while the Hindus blamed the Muslims. This name calling of pandemic disease was also noted during President Trump's period as president of the United States.

In 1492, Ferdinand de Aragon and Isabel of Castilla issued the Alhambra Decree, stating that all Jews convert to Catholicism or be expelled from Spain and its territories. Over half of Spain's Jews had already converted to Catholicism as a result of religious persecution in 1391. As a result of the Alhambra decree and the prior persecution, over 200,000 Jews converted to Catholicism and between 40,000 and 100,000 were expelled. However, it is thought that possibly as many as 200.000 Jews left during the new pogrom for Northern Africa and Southern Europe. On their way, they apparently passed the gates of Rome, despite being forbidden to enter the city. They were subsequently blamed for causing an outbreak of syphilis there that killed at least 30,000 people. Consequently, Jews got blamed for spreading me all over Europe.

These Edicts of Jewish Expulsion began in England as a result of a royal decree issued by King Edward I of England on 18 July 1290. He advised the county sheriffs; he wanted all Jews expelled by no later than All Saints' Day that year. The expulsion edict remained in force for the rest of the Middle Ages. The first Jewish communities of significant size came to England with William the Conqueror in 1066. The Catholic Church strictly forbade the lending of money for profit, and this is why Jews filled that role because of extreme discrimination in every other economic area. Their enterprise ironically led to the building of some of Europe's finest cathedrals and churches, especially under the Medici, an Italian banking family and political dynasty that first began to gather prominence under Cosimo de' Medici in the Republic of Florence during the first half of the 15th century.

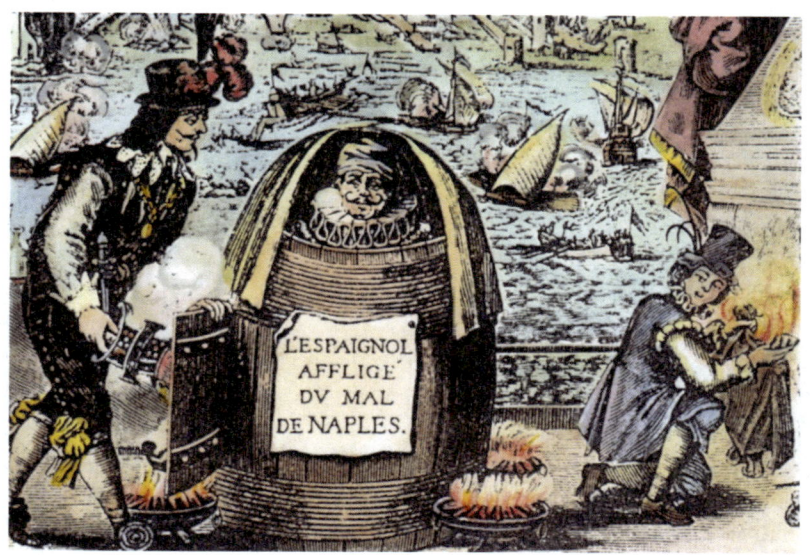

17th CENTURY. Spanish soldier being treated for syphilis (a.k.a. 'Naples disease'),

The causative organism, *Treponema pallidum*, was first identified by German zoologist Fritz Schaudinn and Erich Hoffmann, in 1905. Hoffmann studied medicine at the Berlin Military Academy and was later a professor at the Universities of Halle and Bonn. They discovered a spiral-shaped spirochete on a sample papula removed from the vulva of a patient with secondary syphilis and called me *Treponema pallidum*.

Since the 1490s, the treatment of syphilis has consisted of heavy metals--first mercurial and later arsenic and bismuth preparations. Abraham Colles first described the Colles fracture in 1814, as an extra-articular break of distal radius was the first to introduce mercury therapy for the treatment of syphilis, which was prevalent in the Dublin of the period. He also noted that a child born with the disease tends to infect the healthiest nurse but never its mother. In 1852, Duchenne described tabes dorsalis (syphilis in the third chronic stage) as having various neurologic symptoms as well as sudden stabbing pains followed by vomiting and diarrhoea. These gastric symptoms were probably related to poisoning by heavy metals, including mercury, which produce similar pain reactions and tabes-like neurologic symptoms. By 1875, physicians recognised that some diseases (cholera, diphtheria, scarlet fever, childbirth fever, syphilis, smallpox) were accompanied by specific microorganisms, but the body of medical opinion was unwilling to concede that important diseases could be caused by such agents.

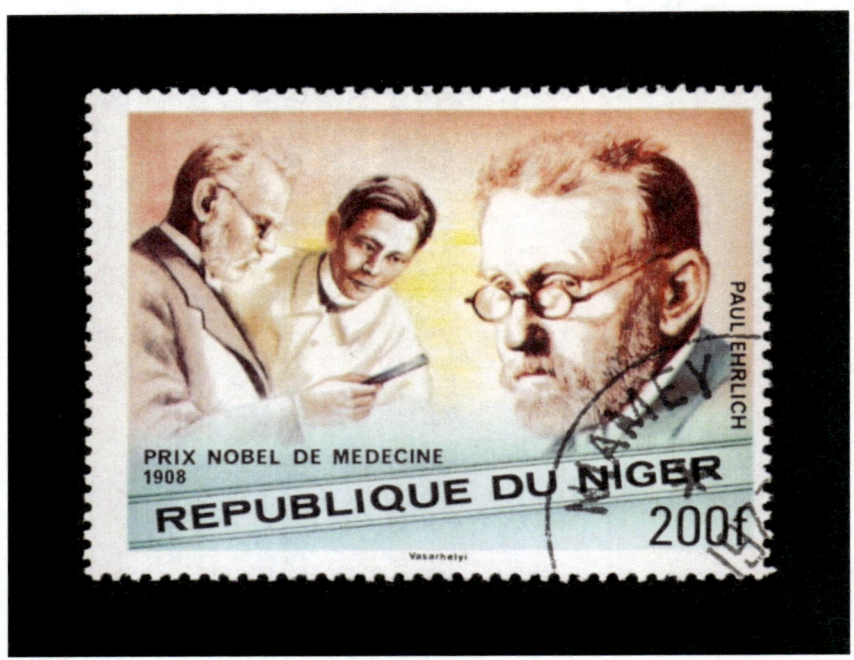

Postage stamp from Niger depicting Paul Ehrlich, discoverer of a cure for syphilis

In 1854, Paul Ehrlich was born in Strehlen, Upper Silesia, Germany, the same year that Florence Nightingale stepped ashore in the mud of Scutari at the start of the Crimean War. In 1882, he became titular professor and later associate professor to the Charité Hospital in Berlin. In 1897, he was appointed public health officer at Frankfurt-am-Main and in 1899, he became the director of the Royal Institute of Experimental Therapy, devoting himself to the emerging science of chemotherapy, hoping to find chemical substances which would have special affinities for pathogenic organisms. He was also the first to use the term 'magic bullets' to describe toxins that would go straight to the organisms at which they were aimed. With the help of his assistants, Ehrlich tested hundreds of chemical substances, hoping to find a magic bullet to treat trypanosomiasis and the other protozoal diseases. He eventually discovered trypan red, which was, as his Japanese assistant Shiga showed, effective against trypanosomes.

Among the arsenical drugs already tested for other purposes was number 606, a substance, which had been set aside in 1907 as being ineffective. One of his research assistants, a prominent Japanese bacteriologist called Sahachiro Hata who had researched the bubonic plague found it to be effective on rabbits infected with syphilis. In 1909, the first effective treatment for syphilis was released. It was called Arsphenamine and was manufactured under the trade name Salvarsan by Hoechst AG. Ehrlich called the substance salvarsan (meaning 'that which saves by arsenic'). The only previous treatments for killing me had been so toxic that they often killed the patient. Further work revealed that another substance, number 914, although less effective, was more easily manufactured and easier to administrate. Ehrlich called this substance, neosalvarsan and he tried to commercialise its use. But he had to battle with much opposition before salvarsan or neosalvarsan was accepted for the treatment of human syphilis.

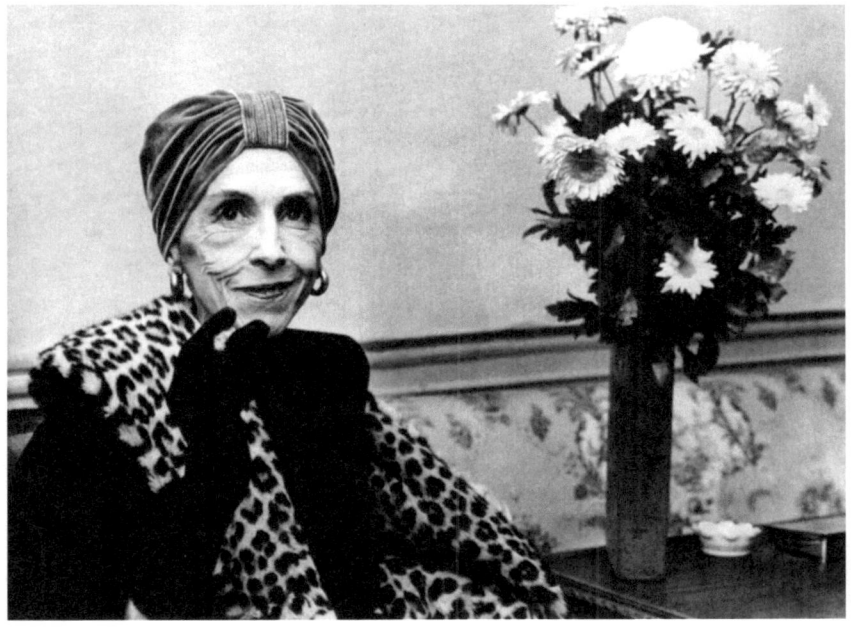

ISAK DINESEN (1885–1962). Pseudonym of Karen Blixen. Danish writer, wearing a fur coat of a leopard she killed while living in Kenya. Photograph, 1959.

Many famous historical figures, including Franz Schubert, Édouard Manet, Karen Blixen and Friedrich Nietzsche are believed to have had the disease. In March 1941, two months after her wedding, Karen Blixen was diagnosed as having syphilis in the second stage. She was treated initially with mercury and later on in Denmark with salvarsan. Friedrich Nietzsche was long believed to have gone mad as a result of tertiary syphilis, but that diagnosis has recently come into question. Karen Blixen got syphilis in 1914 and took mercury pills for a year, after which she experienced severe mercurial intoxication. She received more treatment with mercury, salvarsan, and bismuth, but in fact, her venereologist Carl Rasch told her she was already cured already in 1915. However, she did not believe him, and several specialists in internal medicine and neurology told her many years later that she had to accept the diagnosis *Tabes dorsalis*, i.e., syphilis in the third chronic stage. She had a negative serology, and it is now postulated that her illness was the result of heavy metal poisoning.

Alexander Fleming was born near Darvel in Ayrshire, Scotland in 1881. In 1903, he began studying medicine at St Mary's Paddington, from where he qualified in the same period that Albert Einstein was trying to convince the world that light should be considered as a stream of tiny particles. In 1921, Fleming discovered an important bacteriolytic substance, which he named lysozyme. After returning from a holiday in 1928, he observed the dissolving of staphylococci by a Penicillium mould, and the rest of that story is well-recorded history. Florey and Ernst Chain eventually purified the compound and with them, he was awarded the Nobel Prize in 1945. Alexander Fleming was knighted in 1944 in recognition for his contribution to the development of penicillin. In 1943, penicillin was introduced as a treatment for syphilis by John Mahoney, Richard Arnold, and AD Harris. Large doses of intravenous penicillin G are given for a minimum of 10 days for neurosyphilis, due to the poor penetration of benzathine penicillin into the central nervous system.

In 1908, Erlich shared the Nobel Prize with Ilya Metchnikoff in recognition for their work on immunity. Hata received three unsuccessful nominations for the Nobel Prize in Physiology or Medicine. This organoarsenic compound was the first modern chemotherapy drug. Meanwhile, Alexander Fleming had yet to discover his Penicillin mould, but in London, he developed such a busy practice he got the nickname 'Private 606'. In 2015, about fifty million people worldwide were infected with syphilis. Although the incidence decreased dramatically with the discovery of penicillin in the 1940s, rates of infection have recently increased again in many countries, often in combination with human immunodeficiency virus(HIV).

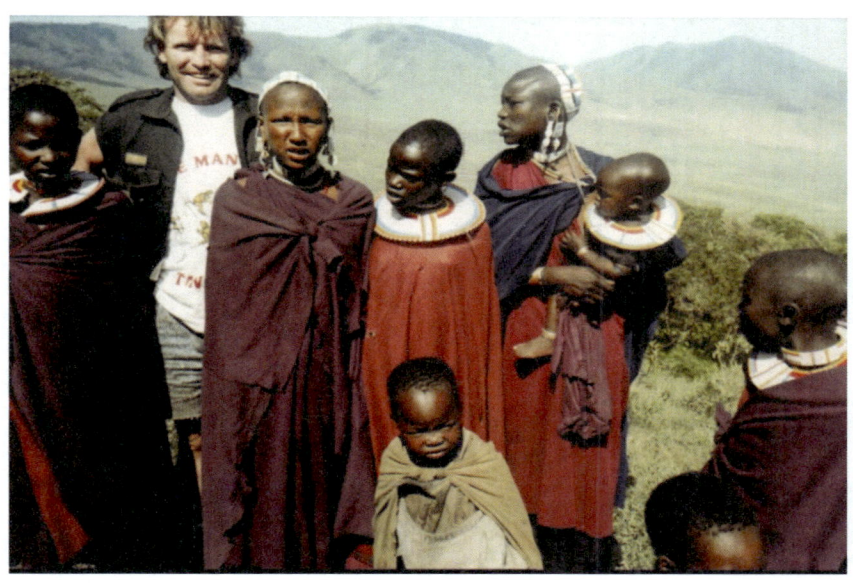

The author with some locals in Kenya in 1992 near Karen Blixen's house, located about 10 km outside of Nairobi at the foot of the Ngong Hills.

I Am *Cocoliztli,* and I Helped Wipe Out the Aztec Civilisation

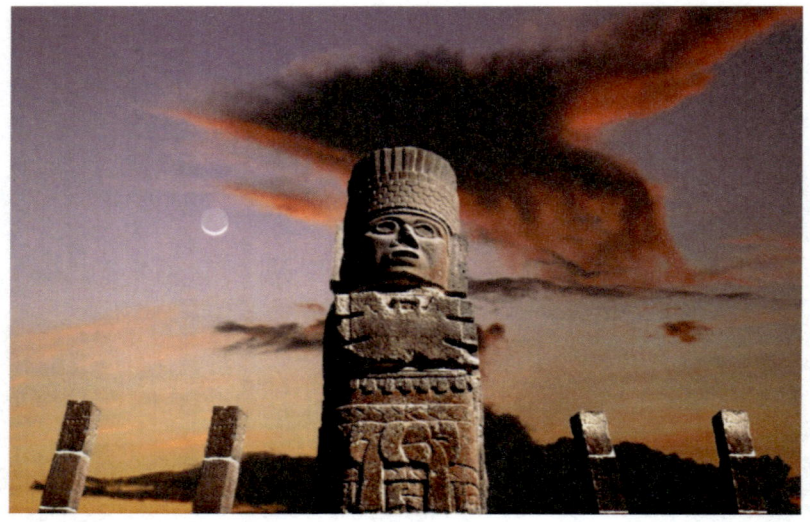

The Atlantes Tula Tolum Mexico

The 1545 and 1576 cocoliztli epidemics appear to have been haemorrhagic fevers caused by an indigenous viral agent and aggravated by unusual climatic conditions. The native people of Mexico experienced an epidemic disease in the wake of European conquest, beginning with the smallpox epidemic of 1519 to 1520 when 5 million to 8 million people perished. The catastrophic epidemics that began in 1545 and 1576 subsequently killed an additional 7 million to 17 million people in the highlands of Mexico. The Mexican population did not recover to pre-Hispanic levels until the 20th century. The Aztecs called it *cocoliztli*, meaning pestilence in the local Nahuatl language. The main victims were Mixtec people, a distinct group from the Aztecs of central Mexico. According to Francisco Hernández de Toledo, a physician who witnessed the outbreak of Cocoliztli in 1576, symptoms included high fever, severe headache, vertigo, black tongue, dark urine, dysentery, severe abdominal and chest pain, head and neck nodules, neurologic disorders, jaundice, and profuse bleeding from the nose, eyes, and mouth. It was a swift and highly lethal disease. Francisco Hernandez was the Proto-Medico of New Spain and former personal physician of King Phillip II. Making him one of the most qualified physicians of the day. He wrote clinical details of symptoms he witnessed amongst the fifteen hundred and eighty cocoliztli infections. The disease described by Dr Hernandez in 1576 is difficult to link to any specific aetiologic agent or disease known today. Some aspects of cocoliztli epidemiology suggest that a native agent hosted in a rain-sensitive rodent reservoir was responsible for the disease. Many of the symptoms described by Dr Hernandez occur to a degree in infections by rodent-borne South American arenaviruses, but no arenavirus has been positively identified in Mexico. Hantavirus is a less likely candidate for cocoliztli because epidemics of severe hantavirus haemorrhagic fevers with high death rates are unknown in the New World. Twenty years before, the Aztec Empire was destroyed by a smallpox infection, the disease killing many of its victims and incapacitating others. It weakened the population, so they were unable to resist Spanish colonizers and left farmers unable to produce needed crops, and now this new disease *cocoliztli* was coming to take the rest. Historical data suggests that approximately 60–70% of the Aztec death toll was caused by a series of epidemics of haemorrhagic fevers of unknown origin. There is some evidence and indicating that the 1545 and 1576 epidemics of cocoliztli (Nahuatl for 'pest') were indigenous haemorrhagic fevers transmitted by rodent hosts and aggravated by extreme drought conditions. The native population collapse in 16th century Mexico was a demographic catastrophe with one of the highest death rates in history.

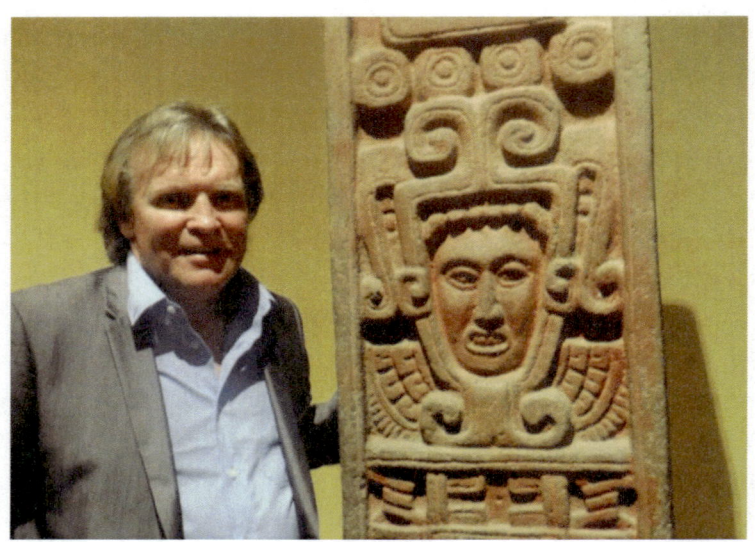

The author in the Aztec Museum Mexico City

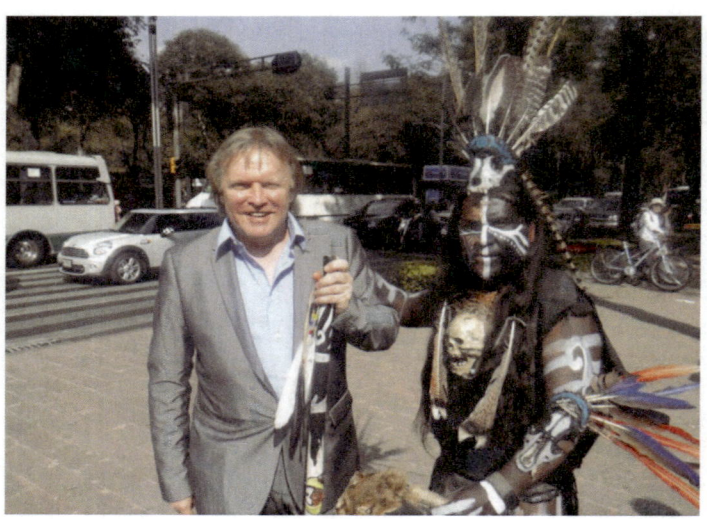

The author with some Mayan natives at Tulum, a town on the coastline of Mexico's Yucatán Peninsula. Tulum, located in the Mexican state of Quintana Roo, is the site of a pre-Columbian Mayan walled city.

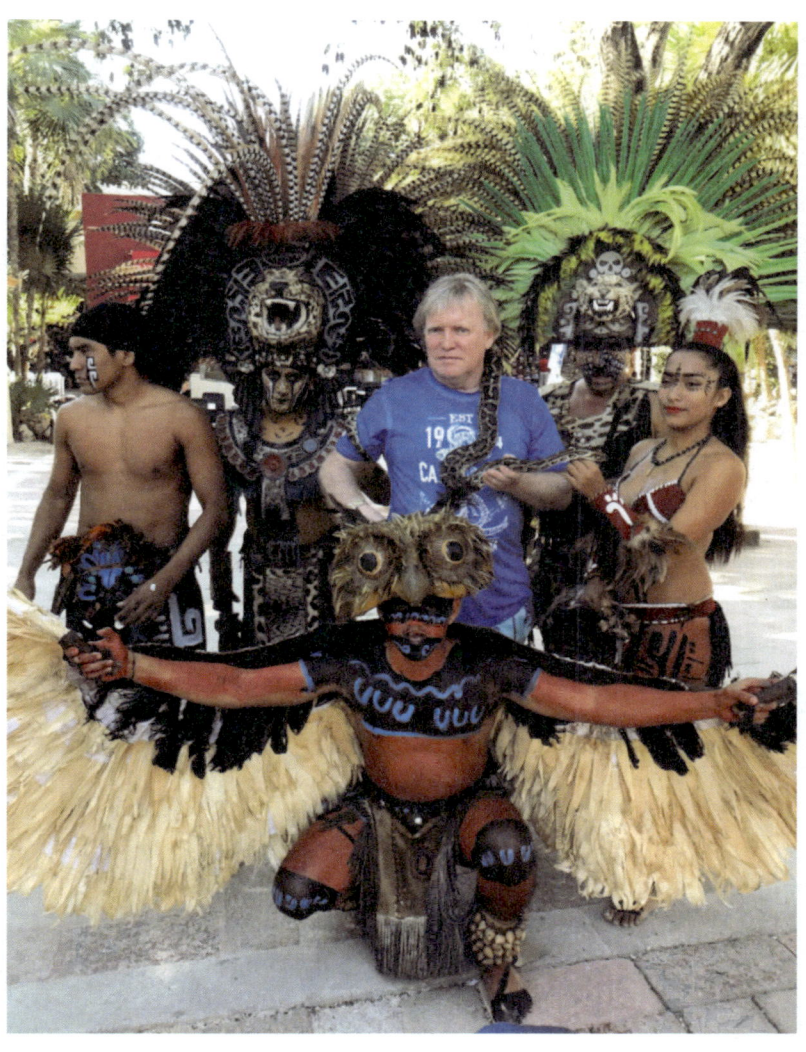

The author with some Mayan natives near Tulum, which served as a major port for Coba, another ancient Mayan city.

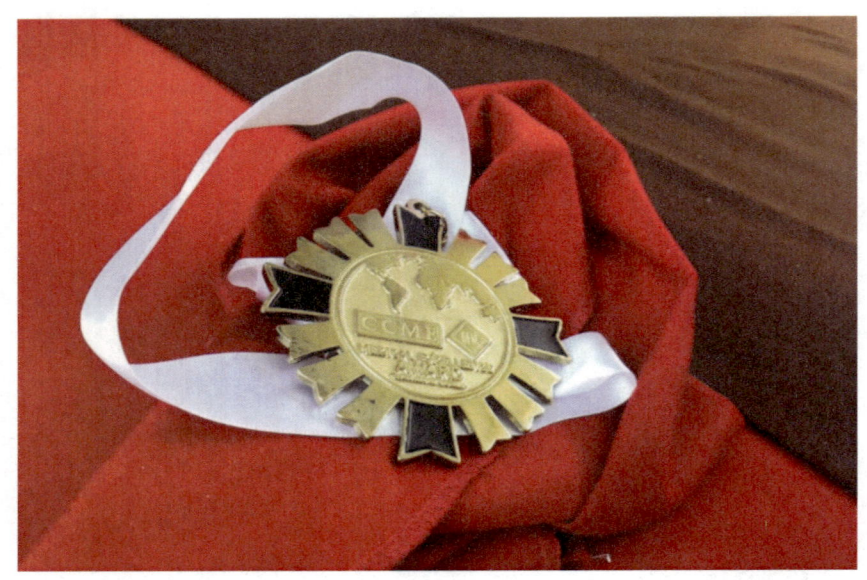

Mexican Medal of Medical Excellence given to the author in 2016

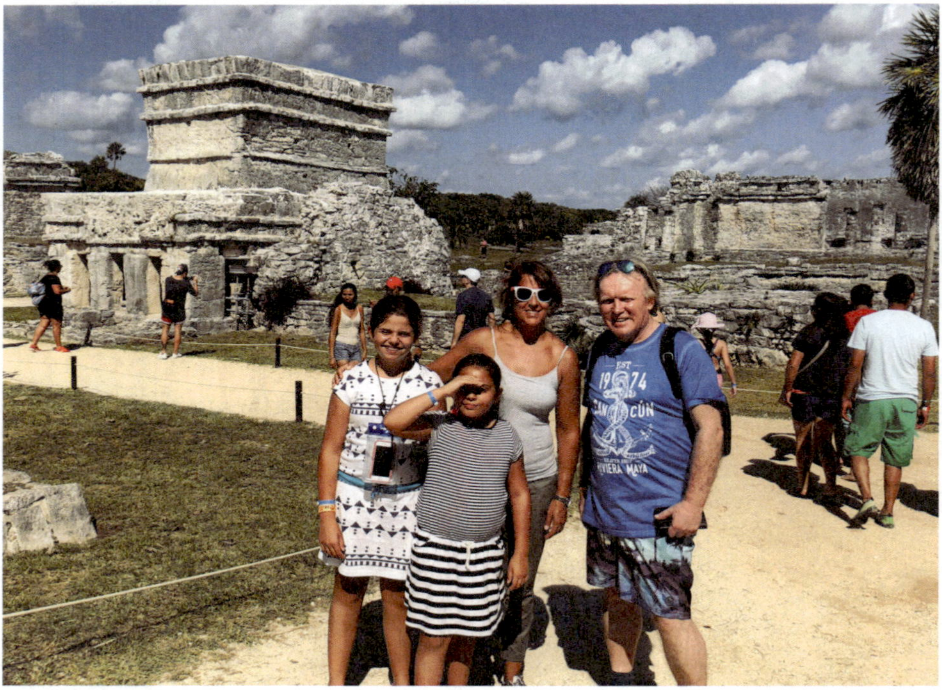

References

Chapter 1 Viruses

1. Lwoff A. The concept of virus. Journal of General Microbiology. 1957;17(2):239–253.
2. Raoult D, Audic S, Robert C, Abergel C, Renesto P, Ogata H, La Scola B, Suzan M, Claverie JM. The 1.2-megabase genome sequence of Mimivirus. Science. 2004;306 (5700):1344–1350.
3. Fraenkel-Conrat H, Singer B. Virus reconstitution. II. Combination of protein and nucleic acid from different strains. Biochimica et Biophysica Acta. 1957;24 (3):540–548.
4. Goldmann DA. Transmission of viral respiratory infections in the home. The Pediatric Infectious Disease Journal. 2000;19 (10 Suppl):S97–S102.
5. Hall CB, Douglas RG, Jr, Geiman JM. Possible transmission by fomites of respiratory syncytial virus. Journal of Infectious Diseases. 1980;141(1):98–102. doi: 10.1093/infdis/141.1.98.
6. Wu KJ (15 April 2020). There are more viruses than stars in the universe. Why do only some infect us? – More than a quadrillion quadrillion individual viruses exist on Earth, but most are not poised to hop into humans. Can we find the ones that are? National Geographic Society. Retrieved 18 May 2020.
7. Koonin EV, Senkevich TG, Dolja VV (September 2006). The ancient Virus World and evolution of cells. Biology Direct. 1 (1):29.
8. Zimmer C (26 February 2021). The Secret Life of a Coronavirus – An oily, 100-nanometer-wide bubble of genes has killed more than two million people and reshaped the world. Scientists don't quite know what to make of it. Dimmock p. 4.
9. Virus Taxonomy: 2019 Release. talk.ictvonline.org. International Committee on Taxonomy of Viruses. Retrieved 25 April 2020.

10. Breitbart M, Rohwer F (June 2005). Here a virus, there a virus, everywhere the same virus? Trends in Microbiology. 13 (6):278–84.
11. Lawrence CM, Menon S, Eilers BJ, Bothner B, Khayat R, Douglas T, Young MJ (May 2009). Structural and functional studies of archaeal viruses. The Journal of Biological Chemistry. 284 (19):12599–603.

Chapter 2 Polio

12. Bodian D, Horstmann DM. Polioviruses. In: Horsfall FL, Tamm I, eds. Viral and Rickettsial infections of Man. 4th ed. Philadelphia, PA: JB Lippincott Co;1965:430–473.
13. Melnick JL. Current status of poliovirus infections. Clin Microbiol Rev. 1996;9(3):293–300.
14. Daniel TM, Robbins FC, eds. A history of poliomyelitis. Polio. Rochester, New York: University of Rochester Press; 1997:5–22.
15. Poliomyelitis. http://www.newworldencyclopedia.org/entry/Poliomyelitis.
16. Trevelyan B, Smallman-Raynor M, Cliff A. The spatial dynamics of poliomyelitis in the United States: from epidemic emergence to vaccine-induced retreat, 1910–1971. Ann Assoc Am Geogr. 2005;95(2):269–293.
17. CDC. The global polio eradication initiative stops transmission of polio (STOP) program—1999–2013. MMWR Morb Mortal Wkly Rep. 2013;62(24):501–503.
18. National Museum of American History. Polio: two vaccines. http://amhistory.si.edu/polio/virusvaccine/vacraces2.html. Accessed November 24, 2013.

Chapter 3 Yellow Fever

19. Reed W, Carroll J, Agramonte A. The etiology of yellow fever: an additional note. JAMA. 1901;36:431–440.
20. Carter HR. Yellow Fever: An Epidemiological and Historical Study of Its Place of Origin. Baltimore, MD: Williams & Wilkins; 1931.

21. Bryan CS, Moss SW, Kahn RJ. Yellow fever in the Americas. Infect Dis Clin North Am. 2004;18(2):275–292.
22. Strode GK, ed, Bugher JC, ed, et al. Yellow Fever. New York, NY: McGraw-Hill Book Co; 1951.
23. Haddow AJ. Yellow fever in central Uganda, 1964, part I: historical introduction. Trans R Soc Trop Med Hyg. 1965;59:436–440.
24. Soper FL. The newer epidemiology of yellow fever. Am J Public Health Nations Health. 1937;27(1):1–14.
25. Lindenbach, B. D.; et al. (2007). Flaviviridae: The Viruses and Their Replication. In Knipe, D. M.; P. M. Howley (eds.). Fields Virology (5th ed.). Philadelphia, PA: Lippincott Williams & Wilkins. p. 1101.
26. Sfakianos, Jeffrey; Hecht, Alan (2009). Babcock, Hilary (ed.). West Nile Virus (Curriculum-based juvenile nonfiction). Deadly Diseases & Epidemics. Foreword by David Heymann (2nd ed.). New York: Chelsea House. p. 17. ISBN 978-1-60413-254-0. The yellow fever virus was isolated in 1927.
27. Monath TP. Yellow fever: Victor, Victoria? conqueror, conquest? epidemics and research in the last forty years and prospects for the future. Am J Trop Med Hyg. 1991;45(1):1–4.
28. AJ. Yellow fever in central Uganda, 1964, part I: historical introduction. Trans R Soc Trop Med Hyg. 1965;59:436–440.
29. Germain M, Cornet M, Herve JP, et al. Recent advances in research regarding sylvatic yellow fever in West and Central Africa. Bull Inst Pasteur. 1982;80:315–325.
30. Proc (Bayl Univ Med Cent). 2000 Jan;13(1):45–49. Benjamin Rush, MD: assassin or beloved healer?
31. Yellow fever Fact sheet N°100". World Health Organization. May 2013. Archived from the original on 19 February 2014.
32. Tolle MA (April 2009). Mosquito-borne diseases. Curr Probl Pediatr Adolesc Health Care. 39(4):97–140.
33. Theiler M, Downs WG. The Arthropod-Borne Viruses of Vertebrates: An Account of the Rockefeller Foundation Virus Program, 1951–1970. London, UK: Yale Press, Ltd; 1973.
34. Monath TP, Cetron MS, Teuwen DE. Yellow fever. In: Plotkin S, Orenstein WA, Offit P, eds. Vaccines. 5th ed. Philadelphia, PA: Saunders Elsevier; 2008:959–1056.

35. Rice CM, Lenches EM, Eddy SR, et al. Nucleotide sequence of yellow fever virus: implications for flavivirus gene expression and evolution. Science. 1985;229(4715):726–730.
36. Lai CJ, Monath TP. Chimeric flaviviruses: novel vaccines against dengue fever, tick-borne encephalitis, and Japanese encephalitis. Adv Virus Res. 2003;61:469–509.
37. World Health Organization. Assessment of yellow fever epidemic risk—a decision-making tool for preventive immunization campaigns. Wkly Epidemiol Rec. 2007;82(18):153–160.
38. Gubler DJ. The changing epidemiology of yellow fever and dengue, 1900 to 2003: full circle? Comp Immunol Microbiol Infect Dis. 2004;27(5):319–330.
39. World Health Organization. Global tuberculosis report 2016. Source: World Health Organization.

Chapter 5 Smallpox

40. Dixon, C. W. 1962. Smallpox. J. & A. Churchill, London.
41. Rhazes. 1848 (Reprint). A treatise on smallpox and measles (translated by Greenhill). Syndenham Society, London.
42. Humphrey, J. H., and R. G. White. 1970. Immunology for students of medicine, 3rd ed. F. A. Davis, Philadelphia.
43. World Health Organization. 1980. The global eradication of smallpox. Final report of the Global Commission for the Certification of Smallpox Eradication. World Health Organization, Geneva.
44. Arita, I. 1980. How technology contributed to the success of global smallpox eradication. W.H.O. Chron.34:175–177.
45. Baron, J. 1838. Life of Dr. Jenner. William Collins & Co., London.
46. Baxby, D. 1979. Edward Jenner, William Woodville, and the origins of vaccinia virus. J. Hist. Med. Appl. Sci.34:134–162.
47. Bowers, J. Z. 1981. The odyssey of smallpox vaccination. Bull. Hist. Med. 55:17–33.
48. Cho, C. T., and H. A. Wenner. 1973. Monkeypox virus. Bacteriol. Rev. 37:1–18.

49. Dumbell, K. R., and D. G. Wells. 1982. The pathogenicity of variola virus. A comparison of the growth of standard strains of variola major and variola minor in cell cultures from human embryos. J. Hyg. 89:389–397.
50. Koplow, David A. (2003). Smallpox: the fight to eradicate a global scourge. Berkeley: University of California Press. ISBN 978-0-520-24220-3.
51. Fisk, D. 1959. Dr. Jenner of Berkeley. W. Heineman, London.
52. Foege, W. H., J. D. Millar, and J. M. Lane. 1971. Selective epidemiologic control in smallpox eradication. Am. J. Epidemiol. 94:311–315.
53. Toxicon 1994 Nov;32(11):1295–304. The life and viper of Dr Patrick Russell MD FRS (1727–1805): physician and naturalist B J Hawgood.
54. J Med Biogr 2001 Feb;9(1):1–6 Alexander Russell (1715–1768) and Patrick Russell (1727–1805): physicians and natural historians of Aleppo B J Hawgood.
55. Stefan Riedel, Edward Jenner and the History of Smallpox and Vaccination, Baylor University Medical Center Proceedings, 18:1, (2005), 22.
56. Shawn Buhr, To Inoculate or Not to Inoculate? The Debate and the Smallpox Epidemic of Boston in 1721, Constructing the Past, 1:1, (2000), 63.
57. William Douglass, A Summary, Historical and Political, of the first Planting Progressive Improvements, and present State of the British Settlements in North America, (Boston: Rogers and Fowle, 1749).
58. Jenner, Edward (1749–1823). rcpe.ac.uk. Royal College of Physicians of Edinburgh. Retrieved 26 June 2018.
59. Riedel, Stefan (January 2005). Edward Jenner and the history of smallpox and vaccination. Proceedings (Baylor University. Medical Center). Baylor University Medical Center. 18(1):21–25.
60. Baxby, Derrick. Jenner, Edward (1749–1823). Oxford Dictionary of National Biography. Oxford University Press. Retrieved 14 February 2014.
61. Baxby, Derrick (1999). Edward Jenner's Inquiry; a bicentenary analysis. Vaccine. 17(4):301–7.
62. Edward Jenner biography. Grand Lodge of British Columbia and Yukon A.F. & A. M.

63. How did Edward Jenner test his smallpox vaccine? Telegraph Media Group.
64. History – Edward Jenner (1749–1823). BBC. 1 November 2006.
65. About Edward Jenner. The Jenner Institute. Retrieved 12 April 2020.
66. Young Edward Jenner, Born in Berkeley. Edward Jenner Museum. Archived from the original on 14 September 2012. Retrieved 4 September 2012.
67. Loncarek K (April 2009). Revolution or reformation. Croatian Medical Journal.
68. George Pearson, ed., An Inquiry Concerning the History of the Cowpox, principally with a View to Supersede and Extinguish the Smallpox (London, England: J. Johnson, 1798).
69. Hammarsten J. F.; et al. (1979). Who discovered smallpox vaccination? Edward Jenner or Benjamin Jesty? Transactions of the American Clinical and Climatological Association. 90:44–55.
70. Rich, E. E.; Johnson, A. M. (1952). The Canadian Historical Review. London: The Hudson's Bay Record Society.
71. Sicker, Martin (2000). The Struggle over the Euphrates Frontier. The Pre-Islamic Middle East. Greenwood. p. 169. ISBN 0-275-96890-1.
72. Eutropius XXXI, 6.24.
73. Smith, Christine A. (1996). Plague in the Ancient World. The Student Historical Journal.
74. Quoted in Tzvetan Todorov, The Conquest of America: The Question of the Other (1999:136).
75. The War Against Smallpox. Strategypage.com (2007-09-25). Retrieved on 2011-12-06.
76. Caspar Henderson (2013-04-10). The Book of Barely Imagined Beings: A 21st Century Bestiary. University of Chicago Press. pp. 20–. ISBN 978-0-226-04470-5.

Chapter 6 Ebola

77. Ebola virus disease, Fact sheet N°103, Updated September 2014. World Health Organization (WHO). September 2014.
78. Dixon MG, Schafer IJ (June 2014). Ebola viral disease outbreak—West Africa, 2014.

79. Filoviridae: Current Taxonomy (2015). International Committee on Taxonomy of Viruses. 2015.
80. Schoepp, Randal J.; Olinger, Gene G. (2014). Chapter 7: Filoviruses. In Liu, Dongyou (ed.). Manual of Security Sensitive Microbes and Toxins. CRC Press.
81. WHO Ebola Response Team (23 September 2014). Ebola virus disease in West Africa – the first 9 months of the epidemic and forward projections. New England Journal of Medicine. 371 (16): 1481–1495.
82. Hoenen T, Groseth A, Feldmann H (July 2012). Current Ebola vaccines. Expert Opin Biol Ther. 12 (7): 859–72.
83. Scott JT, Sesay FR, Massaquoi TA, Idriss BR, Sahr F, Semple MG (April 2016). Post-Ebola Syndrome, Sierra Leone. Emerging Infectious Diseases. 22(4):641–6.
84. Karesh, W. B. & Noble, E. (2009). The bushmeat trade: Increased opportunities for transmission of zoonotic disease. Mount Sinai Journal of Medicine: A Journal of Translational and Personalized Medicine. 76(5):429–444.
85. Wordsworth, Dot (25 October 2014). How Ebola got its name. The Spectator.
86. Peterson AT, Bauer JT, Mills JN (2004). Ecologic and Geographic Distribution of Filovirus Disease. Emerg. Infect. Dis. 10 (1): 40–47.
87. Ebola haemorrhagic fever in Sudan, 1976 (PDF).
88. Feldmann H, Geisbert TW (March 2011). Ebola haemorrhagic fever. Lancet.
89. 377(9768):849–62.
90. 2014 Ebola Virus Disease (EVD) outbreak in West Africa. World Health Organization (WHO). 21 April 2014.
91. Funk DJ, Kumar A (November 2014). Ebola virus disease: an update for anesthesiologists and intensivists. Can J Anaesth.
92. Transmission. Centers for Disease Control and Prevention (CDC). 17 October 2014.
93. Corti D, Misasi J, Mulangu S, Stanley DA, Kanekiyo M, Wollen S, et al. (March 2016). Protective monotherapy against lethal Ebola virus infection by a potently neutralizing antibody. Science. 351(6279):1339–42.

94. Chan M (September 2014). Ebola virus disease in West Africa – no early end to the outbreak. N Engl J Med. 371(13):1183–85.
95. Weingartl HM, Embury-Hyatt C, Nfon C, Leung A, Smith G, Kobinger G (2012). Transmission of Ebola virus from pigs to non-human primates. Scientific Reports. 2:811.
96. Chowell G, Nishiura H (October 2014). Transmission dynamics and control of Ebola virus disease (EVD): a review. BMC Med. 12(1):196.
97. Hewlett, Barry; Hewlett, Bonnie (2007). Ebola, Culture and Politics: The Anthropology of an Emerging Disease. Cengage Learning. p. 103.
98. Ebola haemorrhagic fever in Zaire, 1976 (PDF). Bull. World Health Organ. 56(2):271–93. 1978.
99. Henao-Restrepo AM, Camacho A, Longini IM, Watson CH, Edmunds WJ, Egger M, et al. (February 2017). Efficacy and effectiveness of an rVSV-vectored vaccine in preventing Ebola virus disease: final results from the Guinea ring vaccination, open-label, cluster-randomised trial (Ebola Ça Suffit!). Lancet. 389 (10068): 505–18.
100. Final trial results confirm Ebola vaccine provides high protection against disease (Press release). World Health Organization. 23 December 2016.

Chapter 7 HIV

101. Cold Spring Harb Perspect Med. 2011 Sep; 1 Origins of HIV and the AIDS Pandemic Paul M. Sharp1 and Beatrice H. Hahn.
102. BMJ. 1989 May 13;298(6683):1267–1268. Origin of HIV. M. O. McClure and T. F. Schulz.
103. Wain-Hobson S, Sonigo P, Danos O, Cole S, Alizon M. Nucleotide sequence of the AIDS virus, LAV. Cell. 1985 Jan;40(1):9–17.
104. Daniel MD, Letvin NL, King NW, Kannagi M, Sehgal PK, Hunt RD, Kanki PJ, Essex M, Desrosiers RC. Isolation of T-cell tropic HTLV-III-like retrovirus from macaques. Science. 1985 Jun 7;228(4704):1201–1204.
105. Kestler HW, 3rd, Li Y, Naidu YM, Butler CV, Ochs MF, Jaenel G, King NW, Daniel MD, Desrosiers RC. Comparison of simian

immunodeficiency virus isolates. Nature. 1988 Feb 18;331(6157):619–622.
106. Murphey-Corb M, Martin LN, Rangan SR, Baskin GB, Gormus BJ, Wolf RH, Andes WA, West M, Montelaro RC. Isolation of an HTLV-III-related retrovirus from macaques with simian AIDS and its possible origin in asymptomatic mangabeys. Nature. 1986 May 22;321(6068):435–437.
107. Frøland SS, Jenum P, Lindboe CF, Wefring KW, Linnestad PJ, Böhmer T. HIV-1 infection in Norwegian family before 1970. Lancet. 1988 Jun 11;1(8598):1344–1345.
108. Kawamura M, Yamazaki S, Ishikawa K, Kwofie TB, Tsujimoto H, Hayami M. HIV-2 in west Africa in 1966. Lancet. 1989 Feb 18;1(8634):385–385.
109. Worobey, M. et al (2010). Island biogeography reveals the deep history of SIV Science 329(5998):1487.
110. Sharp, P.M. & Hahn, B.H. (2011). Origins of HIV and the AIDS pandemic Cold Spring Harbour Perspectives in Medicine 1(1):a006841.
111. Gao, F. et al (1999) Origin of HIV-1 in the chimpanzee Pan troglodytes. Nature 397(6718):436–441.
112. Bailes, E. et al (2003) Hybrid Origin of SIV in Chimpanzees Science 300(5626):1713.
113. Sharp, P.M. and Hahn, B.H. (2011). Origins of HIV and the AIDS pandemic, Cold Spring Harbour Perspectives in Medicine 1(1): a006841.
114. Sharp, P.M. & Hahn, B.H. (2011). Origins of HIV and the AIDS pandemic. Cold Spring Harbour Perspectives in Medicine 1(1): a006841.
115. Faria, N.R. et al (2014). The early spread and epidemic ignition of HIV-1 in human populations. Science 346(6205):56–61.
116. Fukasawa M, Miura T, Hasegawa A, Morikawa S, Tsujimoto H, Miki K, Kitamura T, Hayami M. Sequence of simian immunodeficiency virus from African green monkey, a new member of the HIV/SIV group. Nature. 1988 Jun 2;333(6172):457–461.
117. Daniel MD, Li Y, Naidu YM, Durda PJ, Schmidt DK, Troup CD, Silva DP, MacKey JJ, Kestler HW, 3rd, Sehgal PK, et al. Simian

immunodeficiency virus from African green monkeys. J Virol. 1988 Nov;62(11):4123–4128.
118. Toh H, Miyata T. Is the AIDS virus recombinant? Nature. 1985 Jul 4;316(6023):21–22.
119. Faria, N.R. et al (2014). The early spread and epidemic ignition of HIV-1 in human populations. Science 346(6205):56–61.
120. University of Oxford News (2014, 3 October). HIV pandemic's origins located.
121. Hymes, K.B. et al (1981). Kaposi's sarcoma in homosexual men: A report of eight cases. Lancet 2(8247):598–60.
122. Centers for Disease Control (CDC) (1981, 4 July). Kaposi's Sarcoma and Pneumocystis Pneumonia among Homosexual Men – New York City and California. MMWR Weekly 30(4):305–308.
123. Brennan, R.O. & Durack, D.T. (1981). Gay compromise syndrome. Lancet (8259):1338–1339.
124. Centers for Disease Control (CDC) (1982, 9 July). Opportunistic infections and Kaposi's Sarcoma among Haitians in the United States. 31(26):353–4, 360–1.
125. Centers for Disease Control (CDC) (1982, 16 July). Epidemiologic notes and Reports Pneumocystis carinii Pneumonia among persons with hemophilia A. MMWR Weekly 31(27):365–367.
126. Centers for Disease Control (CDC) (1982, 24 September). Current Trends Update on Acquired Immune Deficiency Syndrome (AIDS)—United States. MMWR Weekly 31(37):507–508, 513–514.
127. Farmer, P. (1992) AIDS and Accusation: Haiti and the Geography of Blame. University of California Press.
128. Chen, Z. et al (1997). Human Immunodeficiency Virus Type 2 (HIV-2) Seroprevalence and Characterization of a Distinct HIV-2 Genetic Subtype from the Natural Range of Simian Immunodeficiency Virus-Infected Sooty Mangabeys. Journal of Virology 71(5):3953–3960.
129. Sharp, P.M. & Hahn, B.H. (2011). Origins of HIV and the AIDS pandemic. Cold Spring Harbour Perspectives in Medicine 1(1):a00684.
130. Science (1998). Oldest Surviving HIV Virus Tells All (accessed 11/01/2016.

131. Fara, N.R. et al (2014). The early spread and epidemic ignition of HIV-1 in human populations. Science 346(6205):56–6.

132. BBC News (2014, 3 October). Aids: Origin of pandemic was 1920s Kinshasa.

133. Haiti. www.unaids.org.

134. Fawzi, M.C. Smith; Lambert, W.; Boehm, F.; Finkelstein, Singler, Léandre, F.; Nevil, P.; Bertrand, D.; Claude, (2010-04-10). Economic Risk Factors for HIV Infection Among Women in Rural Haiti: Implications for HIV Prevention Policies and Programs in Resource-Poor Settings. Journal of Women's Health. 19(5):885–892.

135. Dorjgochoo, Tsogzolmaa; Noel, Francine; Deschamps, Marie Marcelle; Theodore, Harry; Dupont, William; Wright, Peter F; Fitzgerald, Dan W; Vermund, Sten H; Pape, Jean W (2009). Risk Factors for HIV Infection Among Haitian Adolescents and Young Adults Seeking Counseling and Testing in Port-au-Prince. Journal of Acquired Immune Deficiency Syndromes. 52(4):498–508.

136. Fridman-Klein AE, Laubenstein LJ, Rubinstein P, Buimovici-Klein E, Marmor M, Stahl R, Spigland I, Kim KS, Zolla-Pazner S. Disseminated Kaposi's sarcoma in homosexual men. Ann Intern Med. 1982 Jun;96(6 Pt 1):693–700.

137. Hui DSC, Zumla A. Severe Acute Respiratory Syndrome: Historical.

Chapter 8 Covid 19

138. Epidemiologic, and Clinical Features. Infect Dis Clin North Am. 2019 Dec;33(4):869–889.

139. Azhar EI, Hui DSC, Memish ZA, Drosten C, Zumla A. The Middle East Respiratory Syndrome (MERS). Infect Dis Clin North Am. 2019 Dec;33(4):891–905. [PMC free article] [PubMed].

140. Perlman S, Netland J. Coronaviruses post-SARS: update on replication and pathogenesis. Nat Rev Microbiol. 2009 Jun;7(6):439–50. [PMC free article] [PubMed].

141. Flaxman S, Mishra S, Gandy A, Unwin HJT, Mellan TA, Coupland H, Whittaker C, Zhu H, Berah T, Eaton JW, Monod M, Imperial College COVID-19 Response Team. Ghani AC, Donnelly CA,

Riley S, Vollmer MAC, Ferguson NM, Okell LC, Bhatt S. Estimating the effects of non-pharmaceutical interventions on COVID-19 in Europe. Nature. 2020 Aug;584(7820):257–261.
142. Lu R, Zhao X, Li J, Niu P, Yang B, Wu H, et al. Genomic characterisation and epidemiology of 2019 novel coronavirus: implications for virus origins and receptor binding. Lancet. 2020;395(10224):565–74.
143. WHO. Coronavirus disease (COVID-2019) situation reports. 2020. https://www.who.int/emergencies/diseases/novel-coronavirus-2019/situation-reports.
144. Riou J, Althaus CL. Pattern of early human-to-human transmission of Wuhan 2019 novel coronavirus (2019-nCoV), December 2019 to January 2020. Euro Surveill. 2020;25(4):2000058. https://doi.org/10.2807/1560-7917.ES.2020.25.4.2000058.
145. Liu Y, Gayle AA, Wilder-Smith A, Rocklov J. The reproductive number of COVID-19 is higher compared to SARS coronavirus. J Travel Med. 2020. https://doi.org/10.1093/jtm/taaa021.
146. Chan JF, Yuan S, Kok KH, To KK, Chu H, Yang J, et al. A familial cluster of pneumonia associated with the 2019 novel coronavirus indicating person-to-person transmission: a study of a family cluster. Lancet. 2020;395(10223):514–23.
147. Dhama K, Sharun K, Tiwari R, Dadar M, Malik YS, Singh KP & Chaicumpa W (2020). COVID-19, an emerging coronavirus infection: advances and prospects in designing and developing vaccines, immunotherapeutics, and therapeutics. Hum Vaccin Immunother, 1–7. https://doi.org/10.1080/21645515.2020.1735227.
148. Wu R, Wang L, Kuo HD, Shannar A, Peter R, Chou PJ, Li S, Hudlikar R, Liu X, Liu Z, et al. (2020). An update on current therapeutic drugs treating COVID-19. Curr Pharmacol Rep, 1–15. https://doi.org/10.1007/s40495-020-00216-7.
149. GlebovOO (2020). Understanding SARS-CoV-2 endocytosis for COVID-19 drug repurposing. FEBS J 287, 3664–3671.
150. Atzrodt CL, Maknojia I, McCarthy RDP, Oldfield TM, Po J, Ta KTL, Stepp HE & Clements TP (2020). A Guide to COVID-19: a global pandemic caused by the novel coronavirus SARS-CoV-2. FEBS J 287, 3633–3650.

151. Sharpe HR, Gilbride C, Allen E, Belij-Rammerstorfer S, Bissett C, Ewer K & Lambe T (2020). The early landscape of COVID-19 vaccine development in the UK and rest of the world. Immunology. https://doi.org/10.1111/imm.13222.

152. Nitulescu G, Paunescu H, Moschos S, Petrakis D, Nitulescu G, Ion G, Spandidos D, Nikolouzakis T, Drakoulis N & Tsatsakis A (2020). Comprehensive analysis of drugs to treat SARS-CoV-2 infection: Mechanistic insights into current COVID-19 therapies (Review). Int J Mol Med. https://doi.org/10.3892/ijmm.2020.4608.

153. Febs Journal COVID-19 breakthroughs: separating fact from fiction, Paraminder Dhillon Manuel Breuer Natasha Hirst Volume 287, Issue17 Focus Issue: COVID-19 September 2020, Pages 3612–3632 First published: 05 June 2020 https://doi.org/10.1111/febs.15442.

154. World Health Organization (2020). Novel Coronavirus (2019-nCoV) Situation Report-1. https://www.who.int/docs/default-source/coronaviruse/situation-reports/20200121-sitrep-1-2019-ncov.pdf.

155. Guan Y, Zheng BJ, He YQ, Liu XL, Zhuang ZX, Cheung CL, Luo SW, Li PH, Zhang LJ, Guan YJ, et al. (2003). Isolation and characterization of viruses related to the SARS coronavirus from animals in southern China. Science 302(5643): 276–278.

156. Huang C, Wang Y, Li X, Ren L, Zhao J, Hu Y, Zhang L, Fan G, Xu J, Gu X, et al. (2020). Clinical features of patients infected with 2019 novel coronavirus in Wuhan, China. Lancet 395(10223): 497–506.

157. Li Q, Guan X, Wu P, Wang X, Zhou L, Tong Y, Ren R, Leung KSM, Lau EHY, Wong JY, et al. (2020). Early transmission dynamics in Wuhan, China, of novel coronavirus-infected pneumonia. N Engl J Med 382, 1199–1207.

158. Sky News (2020) Coronavirus: Mike Pompeo says 'significant evidence' COVID-19 came from Wuhan lab. https://news.sky.com/story/coronavirus-mike-pompeo-says-significant-evidence-covid-19-came-from-wuhan-lab-11982686.

159. Sky News (2020) Coronavirus: Mike Pompeo says 'significant evidence' COVID-19 came from Wuhan lab. https://news.sky.com/story/coronavirus-mike-pompeo-says-significant-evidence-covid-19-came-from-wuhan-lab-11982686.

160. Bast F (2020). A Nobel Laureate Said the New Coronavirus Was Made in a Lab. He's Wrong. https://sciencethewirein/the-sciences/luc-montagnier-coronavirus-wuhan-lab-pseudoscience.

161. Pradhan P, Pandey AK, Mishra A, Gupta P, Tripathi PK, Menon MB, Gomes J, Vivekanandan P & Kundu B (2020). Uncanny similarity of unique inserts in the 2019-nCoV spike protein to HIV-1 gp120 and Gag. bioRxiv. "[PREPRINT]".

162. Xiao C, Li X, Liu S, Sang Y, Gao SJ & Gao F (2020). HIV-1 did not contribute to the 2019-nCoV genome. Emerg Microbes Infect 9, 378–381.

163. Andersen KG, Rambaut A, Lipkin WI, Holmes EC & Garry RF (2020). The proximal origin of SARS-CoV-2. Nat Med 26, 450–452.

164. Hoffmann M, Kleine-Weber H, Schroeder S, Kruger N, Herrler T, Erichsen S, Schiergens TS, Herrler G, Wu NH, Nitsche A, et al. (2020). SARS-CoV-2 cell entry depends on ACE2 and TMPRSS2 and is blocked by a clinically proven protease inhibitor. Cell 181, 271–280.e8.

165. PUBPEER (2020). The proximal origin of SARS-CoV2.

166. HoffmannM, Kleine-WeberH, SchroederS, KrugerN, HerrlerT, ErichsenS, SchiergensTS, HerrlerG, WuNH, NitscheAet al. (2020). SARS-CoV-2 cell entry depends on ACE2 and TMPRSS2 and is blocked by a clinically proven protease inhibitor. Cell 181, 271–280.e8.

167. PUBPEER (2020). The proximal origin of SARS-CoV2. https://pubpeer.com/publications/E3130C13E4C47CB08296D195CF47B9.

168. Zhou P, Yang XL, Wang XG, Hu B, Zhang L, Zhang W, Si HR, Zhu Y, Li B, Huang CL, et al. (2020). A pneumonia outbreak associated with a new coronavirus of probable bat origin. Nature 579, 270–273.

169. Li W, Shi Z, Yu M, Ren W, Smith C, Epstein JH, Wang H, Crameri G, Hu Z, Zhang H, et al. (2005). Bats are natural reservoirs of SARS-like coronaviruses. Science 310, 676–679.

170. Zhu N, Zhang D, Wang W, Li X, Yang B, Song J, Zhao X, Huang B, Shi W, Lu R, et al. (2020). A novel coronavirus from patients with pneumonia in China, 2019. N Engl J Med 382, 727–733.

171. Zhang YZ & Holmes EC (2020). A genomic perspective on the origin and emergence of SARS-CoV-2. Cell 181, 223–227.

172. Wu F, Zhao S, Yu B, Chen YM, Wang W, Song ZG, Hu Y, Tao ZW, Tian JH, Pei YY, et al. (2020). A new coronavirus associated with human respiratory disease in China. Nature 579, 265–269.
173. Zhou H, Chen X, Hu T, Li J, Song H, Liu Y, Wang P, Liu D, Yang J, Holmes EC, et al. (2020). A novel bat coronavirus closely related to SARS-CoV-2 contains natural insertions at the S1/S2 cleavage site of the spike protein. Curr Biol 30, 2196–2203.
174. Wu CN, Xia LZ, Li KH, Ma WH, Yu DN, Qu B, Li BX, Cao Y. High-flow nasal-oxygenation-assisted fibreoptic tracheal intubation in critically ill patients with COVID-19 pneumonia: a prospective randomised controlled trial. Br J Anaesth. 2020 Jul;125(1):e166–e168.
175. Ledford H. Coronavirus breakthrough: dexamethasone is first drug shown to save lives. Nature. 2020 Jun;582(7813):469.
176. Bimonte S, Crispo A, Amore A, Celentano E, Cuomo A, Cascella M. Potential Antiviral Drugs for SARS-Cov-2 Treatment: Preclinical Findings and Ongoing Clinical Research. In Vivo. 2020 Jun;34(3 Suppl):1597–1602.
177. Cao B, Wang Y, Wen D, Liu W, Wang J, Fan G, Ruan L, Song B, Cai Y, Wei M, Li X, Xia J, Chen N, Xiang J, Yu T, Bai T, Xie X, Zhang L, Li C, Yuan Y, Chen H, Li H, Huang H, Tu S, Gong F, Liu Y, Wei Y, Dong C, Zhou F, Gu X, Xu J, Liu Z, Zhang Y, Li H, Shang L, Wang K, Li K, Zhou X, Dong X, Qu Z, Lu S, Hu X, Ruan S, Luo S, Wu J, Peng L, Cheng F, Pan L, Zou J, Jia C, Wang J, Liu X, Wang S, Wu X, Ge Q, He J, Zhan H, Qiu F, Guo L, Huang C, Jaki T, Hayden FG, Horby PW, Zhang D, Wang C. A Trial of Lopinavir-Ritonavir in Adults Hospitalized with Severe Covid-19. N Engl J Med. 2020 May 07;382(19):1787–1799.
178. Gordon CJ, Tchesnokov EP, Feng JY, Porter DP, Götte M. The antiviral compound remdesivir potently inhibits RNA-dependent RNA polymerase from Middle East respiratory syndrome coronavirus. J Biol Chem. 2020 Apr 10;295(15):4773–4779.
179. de Wit E, Feldmann F, Cronin J, Jordan R, Okumura A, Thomas T, Scott D, Cihlar T, Feldmann H. Prophylactic and therapeutic remdesivir (GS-5734) treatment in the rhesus macaque model of MERS-CoV infection. Proc Natl Acad Sci U S A 2020 Mar 24;117(12):6771–6776.

180. Williamson BN, Feldmann F, Schwarz B, Meade-White K, Porter DP, Schulz J, van Doremalen N, Leighton I, Yinda CK, Pérez-Pérez L, Okumura A, Lovaglio J, Hanley PW, Saturday G, Bosio CM, Anzick S, Barbian K, Cihlar T, Martens C, Scott DP, Munster VJ, de Wit E. Clinical benefit of remdesivir in rhesus macaques infected with SARS-CoV-2. Nature. 2020 Sep;585(7824):273–276.

181. Chen N, Zhou M, Dong X, Qu J, Gong F, Han Y, Qiu Y, Wang J, Liu Y, Wei Y, Xia J, Yu T, Zhang X, Zhang L. Epidemiological and clinical characteristics of 99 cases of 2019 novel coronavirus pneumonia in Wuhan, China: a descriptive study. Lancet. 2020 Feb 15;395(10223):507–513.

182. Wang Z, Yang B, Li Q, Wen L, Zhang R. Clinical Features of 69 Cases With Coronavirus Disease 2019 in Wuhan, China. Clin Infect Dis. 2020 Jul 28;71(15):769–777.

183. Gautret P, Lagier JC, Parola P, Hoang VT, Meddeb L, Mailhe M, Doudier B, Courjon J, Giordanengo V, Vieira VE, Tissot Dupont H, Honoré S, Colson P, Chabrière E, La Scola B, Rolain JM, Brouqui P, Raoult D. Hydroxychloroquine and azithromycin as a treatment of COVID-19: results of an open-label non-randomized clinical trial. Int J Antimicrob Agents. 2020 Jul;56(1):105949.

184. Zarogoulidis P, Papanas N, Kioumis I, Chatzaki E, Maltezos E, Zarogoulidis K. Macrolides: from in vitro anti-inflammatory and immunomodulatory properties to clinical practice in respiratory diseases. Eur J Clin Pharmacol. 2012 May;68(5):479–503.

185. Kollias A, Kyriakoulis KG, Dimakakos E, Poulakou G, Stergiou GS, Syrigos K. Thromboembolic risk and anticoagulant therapy in COVID-19 patients: emerging evidence and call for action. Br J Haematol. 2020 Jun;189(5):846–84.

186. Buonaguro FM, Puzanov I, Ascierto PA. Anti-IL6R role in treatment of COVID-19-related ARDS. J Transl Med. 2020 Apr 14;18(1):165.

Chapter 9 Anthrax

187. Frankema E and Tworek H (2020). Pandemics that changed the world: historical reflections on COVID-19. Journal of Global History 15:333–335, doi:10.1017/S1740022820000339.
188. Encyclopedia of Pestilence, Pandemics, and Plagues by Ed, Joseph P. Byrne, published by Greenwood Press, 2008.
189. The Anthrax Cleanup of Capitol Hill. Documentary by Xin Wang produced by the EPA Alumni Association.
190. Fishbein MC. Anthrax – From Russia with Love. Infectious Diseases: Causes, Types, Prevention, Treatment and Facts. MedicineNet.com.
191. Disease and History by Frederick C. Cartwright, published by Sutton Publishing, 2014.
192. Suffin SC, Carnes WH, Kaufmann AF (September 1978). Inhalation anthrax in a home craftsman. Human Pathology. 9(5):594–7.
193. Decker J (2003). Deadly Diseases and Epidemics, Anthrax. Chelsea House Publishers. pp. 27–28.

Chapter 10 Plague of Justinian

194. Epidemics and Society: From the Black Death to the Present Frank M. Snowden Oct 2019 Yale University Press.
195. Arrizabalaga, Jon (2010), Bjork, Robert E. (ed.), "Plague and epidemic", The Oxford Dictionary of the Middle Ages, Oxford University Press.
196. Stathakopoulos, Dionysios (2018), Plague, Justinianic (Early Medieval Pandemic), The Oxford Dictionary of Late Antiquity, Oxford University Press.
197. Cyril A. Mango, Byzantium: The Empire of New Rome (1980) emphasizes the demographic effects; Mark Whittow, Ruling the late Roman and Byzantine city, Past and Present 33 (1990) argues against too great reliance on literary sources.
198. Mordechai, Lee; Eisenberg, Merle (August 1, 2019). Rejecting Catastrophe: The Case of the Justinianic Plague. Past & Present. Oxfordshire, England: Oxford University Press.

199. Dio Cassius, LXXII 14.3–4; his book that would cover the plague under Marcus Aurelius is missing; the later outburst was the greatest of which the historian had knowledge.
200. Reactions to Plague in the Ancient & Medieval World. Ancient History Encyclopedia. Retrieved 2021-02-06.
201. Past pandemics that ravaged Europe. BBC News. November 7, 2005.

Chapter 11 Leprosy

202. Global leprosy situation (2012). Wkly Epidemiol Rec. 2012 Aug 24;87(34):317–28.
203. World Health Organization (2012). Global leprosy situation 2012. Wkly Epidemiol Rec 87:317–328.
204. Woodall P, Scollard D, Rajan L (2011). Hansen's disease among Micronesian and Marshallese persons living in the United States. Emerg Infect Dis 17:1202. doi:10.3201/eid1707.102036.
205. Han XY, Seo YH, Sizer KC, Schoberle T, May GS, Spencer JS, Li W, Nair RG. 2008. A new Mycobacterium species causing diffuse lepromatous leprosy. Am J Clin Pathol 130:856–864.
206. Hansen GHA (1874). Undersøgelser Angående Spedalskhedens Årsager (Investigations concerning the etiology of leprosy). Norsk Mag. Laegervidenskaben (in Norwegian). 4:1–88.
207. Irgens L (2002). The discovery of the leprosy bacillus. Tidsskr Nor Laegeforen. 122 (7): 708–9.
208. Brubaker ML, Meyers WM, Bourland J (1985). Leprosy in children one year of age and under. Int J Lepr Other Mycobact Dis 53:517–523.
209. Kumar BS, Dogra S, Kaur I (2004). Epidemiological characteristics of leprosy reactions: 15 years' experience from north India. Int J Lepr Other Mycobact Dis 72:125–133.
210. William S. Haubrich (2003). Medical Meanings: A Glossary of Word Origins. ACP Press.
211. Michael Wilkins; Craig A. Evans; Darrell Bock; Andreas J. Köstenberger (1 October 2013). The Gospels and Acts. B&H Publishing Group.

212. Encyclopedia of Jewish Medical Ethics: A Compilation of Jewish Medical Law on All Topics of Medical Interest...Feldheim Publishers. 2003. p. 951.
213. Robert I. Rotberg (2001). Population History and the Family: A Journal of Interdisciplinary History Reader. MIT Press. p. 132.
214. Montgomerie, John Z (1988). Leprosy in New Zealand. Journal of the Polynesian Society. 97(2):115–152.

Chapter 12 Tuberculosis

215. Tuberculosis (TB). World Health Organization (WHO). 16 February 2018. Retrieved 15 September 2018.
216. Hawn TR, Day TA, Scriba TJ, Hatherill M, Hanekom WA, Evans TG, et al. (December 2014). Tuberculosis vaccines and prevention of infection. Microbiology and Molecular Biology Reviews. 78(4):650–71.
217. McShane H (October 2011). Tuberculosis vaccines: beyond bacille Calmette-Guerin. Philosophical Transactions of the Royal Society of London. Series B, Biological Sciences. 366(1579):2782–89.
218. Roy A, Eisenhut M, Harris RJ, Rodrigues LC, Sridhar S, Habermann S, et al. (August 2014). Effect of BCG vaccination against Mycobacterium tuberculosis infection in children: systematic review and meta-analysis. BMJ. 349.
219. History: World TB Day. Centers for Disease Control and Prevention (CDC). 12 December 2016.

Chapter 13 Malaria

220. Ramsay, Michael A. E. (6 January 2009). John Snow, MD: anaesthetist to the Queen of England and pioneer epidemiologist. Proceedings (Baylor University. Medical Center). 19(1):24–28.
221. John (1854). The cholera near Golden-Square, and at Deptford. The Medical Times and Gazette. 2nd series. 9: 321–322.
222. Disease: The Story of Disease and Mankind's Continuing Struggle Against It by Mary Dobson, published by Quercus, 2007.

223. Source Book of Medical History, Logan Clendening, published by Dover Publications, 1960.
224. Coatney, G. Robert; Collins, William E.; Warren, McWilson; Contacos, Peter George (1971). Plasmodium vivax (Grassi and Feletti, 1890). The primate malarias. Division of Parasitic Disease, CDC. pp. 43–44.
225. Biology: Malaria Parasites. Malaria. CDC. 2004-04-23. Archived from the original on 2008-10-13. Retrieved 2008-09-30.
226. Health problems of Vietnamese refugee children. J Iowa Med Soc. 1975 Dec;65(12):508–510.

Chapter 14 Cholera

227. Snow, John (1854). The cholera near Golden-Square, and at Deptford. The Medical Times and Gazette. 2nd series. 9: 321–322.
228. Disease: The Story of Disease and Mankind's Continuing Struggle Against It by Mary Dobson, published by Quercus, 2007.
229. Filippo Pacini (1854). Osservazioni microscopiche e deduzioni patologiche sul cholera asiatico (Microscopic observations and pathological deductions on Asiatic cholera), Gazzetta Medica Italiana: Toscana, 2nd series, 4(50):397–401; 4(51):405–412. The term "vibrio cholera" appears on page 411.
230. Real Academia de la Historia, ed. (2018). Joaquín Balcells y Pasqual (in Spanish). Archived from the original on 2019-07-08. Retrieved 2020-08-01.
231. Collegi Oficial de Metges de Barcelona, ed. (2015). Joaquim Balcells i Pascual (in Catalan). Archived from the original on 2020-08-01. Retrieved 2020-08-01.

Chapter 15 Syphilis

232. Hackett CJ. On the origin of the human treponematoses (pinta, yaws, endemis syphilis and venereal syphilis). Bull World Health Organ. 1963; 29:7–41.

233. Clin Infect Dis. 2000 Oct;31(4):936–41. First European exposure to syphilis: the Dominican Republic at the time of Columbian contact B M Rothschild 1, F L Calderon, A Coppa, C Rothschild.
234. Rothschild BM. History of Syphilis. Clinical Infectious Diseases. 2005;40:1454–1463.
235. Fee E. The wages of sin. The Lancet. 1999;354:SIV61.
236. Foa A, compiler. In: The new and the old: the spread of syphilis (1494–1530) Baltimore: Johns Hopkins University Press; 1990. pp. 26–45.
237. Sex Transm Dis. May-Jun 1995;22(3):137–44. Neurosyphilis, or chronic heavy metal poisoning: Karen Blixen's lifelong disease K Weismann.
238. Schaudinn, Fritz Richard; Hoffmann, Erich (1905). "Vorläufiger Bericht über das Vorkommen von Spirochaeten in syphilitischen Krankheitsprodukten und bei Papillomen" [Preliminary report on the occurrence of Spirochaetes in syphilitic chancres and papillomas]. Arbeiten aus dem Kaiserlichen Gesundheitsamte. 22: 527–534.
239. Waugn MA. Role played by Italy in the history of syphilis. Br J Vener Dis. 1982;58:92–95.
240. Forrai J, compiler. In: History of Different Therapeutics of Venereal Disease Before the Discovery of Penicillin, Syphilis Recognition, Description and Diagnosis. Dr. Neuza Satomi Sato; 2011.
241. Morton RS. Another look at the Morbus Gallicus. Postscript to the meeting of the Medical Society for the Study of Venereal Diseases. Br J Vener Dis. 1968;44:174–177.
242. Baker B, Armelagos GJ. The origin and antiquity of syphilis: Paleopathological diagnosis and interpretation. Current Anthropology. 1988;29:703–738.
243. Hudson EH. Treponematosis and African Slavery. Br J Vener Dis. 1964;40:43–52.
244. Harper KN, Zuckerman MK, Harper ML. The origin and antiquity of syphilis revisited: an appraisal of Old World pre-Columbian evidence for treponemal infection. Am J Phys Anthropol. 2011;146:99–133.

245. Armelagos GJ, Zuckerman MK, Harper KN. The Science behind Pre-Columbian Evidence of Syphilis in Europe: Research by Documentary. Evol Anthropol. 2012;21:50–57.

246. Roth N, compiler. In: Conversos, Inquisition, and the Expulsion of the Jews from Spain. University of Wisconsin Press; 2002.

247. Sefton AM. The Great Pox that was...syphilis. Journal of Applied Microbiology. 2001;91:592–596.

Chapter 16 Cocoliztli and Mexico

248. Emerg Infect Dis. 2002 Apr; 8(4):360–362. Megadrought and Megadeath in 16th Century Mexico Rodolfo Acuna-Soto,* David W. Stahle, corresponding author† Malcolm K. Cleaveland,† and Matthew D. Therrell†

249. Cook SF, Simpson LB The Population of Central Mexico in the Sixteenth Century. Ibero Americana Vol. 31, Berkeley: University of California Press; 1948.

250. Gerhard P A guide to the historical geography of New Spain. Norman, OK: University of Oklahoma Press; 1993.

251. Hugh T Conquest, Montezuma, Cortez, and the Fall of Old Mexico. New York: Simon and Schuster; 1993.

252. Acuna-Soto R, Caderon Romero L, Maguire JH Large epidemics of hemorrhagic fevers in Mexico 1545–1815. Am J Trop Med Hyg. 2002.

253. Marr JS, Kiracofe JB Was the Huey Cocoliztli a haemorrhagic fever? Med Hist. 2000;44:341–62.

254. Stahle DW, Cleaveland MK, Therrell MD, Villanueva-Diaz J Tree-ring reconstruction of winter and summer precipitation in Durango, Mexico, for the past 600 years. 10th Symposium Global Change Studies. Boston: American Meteorological Society, 1999; 317–8.